SIMPLE COMMON CASES IN CT SCAN

FOR INTERNS AND NEW RESIDENTS

This page intentionally left blank

SIMPLE COMMON CASES IN CT SCAN

FOR INTERNS AND NEW RESIDENTS

MAHMOUD H. MILAD
Head and Consultant
Department of Radiology
Sebha Medical Center
Associate Professor of Radiology
Faculty of Medicine
University of Sebha
Sebha, Libya

ABDALLA M. GAMAL
Senior House Officer
Department of Radiology
Sebha Medical Center
Sebha, Libya.

2015

Copyright © 2015 by Authors

All rights reserved. This book or any portion thereof may not be reproduced or used in any manner whatsoever without the express written permission of the authors except for the use of brief quotations in a book review or scholarly journal.

First Printing: 2015

ISBN-13: 978-1514709962
ISBN-10: 1514709961

Printed by:
CreateSpace, Charleston SC
United States

Correspondence to:
Abdalla M. Gamal
Radiology Department
Sebha Medical Center
Sebha, Libya.
Telephone number: +218944359166
Email address: abdallamutwakilgamal@gmail.com
Website address: www.abdallagamal.com

DEDICATION

To our families for their continous support and encourgement.

To our patients for everything they taught us.

And To you, the one who is reading this book.

TABLE OF CONTENTS

1. Acute limbs weakness and inability to speak _____ 1
2. Acute left sided weakness _____ 5
3. An old female with loss of conciousness _____ 8
4. Chronic headache and vomiting _____ 11
5. An adult male with convlsions _____ 14
6. An old male with right sided facial palsy _____ 17
7. An incidental intracranial cyst found on head CT _____ 20
8. An infant with large head _____ 23
9. A teenage female with hydrocephalus and shunt _____ 26
10. Hyperdense sulci after a head trauma. _____ 29
11. A drowzy child after head trauma _____ 32
12. An adult male with facial trauma _____ 35
13. An adult male with a blow to the jaw _____ 38
14. Chronic nasal obstruction and congestion _____ 41
15. Progressive nasal stuffiness and facial pain _____ 44
16. Nasal congestion and snoring _____ 47
17. Acute pain in the right ear with hearing impairment _____ 50
18. Slowy growing neck swelling _____ 53
19. Lung cavitations in a 25-year-old male _____ 57
20. Foul smelling sputum after pneumonia _____ 61
21. Fever, night sweats and pleuritic chest pain. _____ 64
22. An old male with a solitary lung nodule _____ 67

23. Chronic cough and shortness of breath_____ 70
24. An incidental subcutaneous mass in the back _____ 73
25. A cystic liver lesion on ultrasound_____ 76
26. An epigastric mass and weight loss_____ 79
27. Acute epigastric pain and vomiting_____ 82
28. Painless obstructive jaundice _____ 85
29. An old man with painless hematuria_____ 89
30. An adult female with Right illiac fossa pain _____ 93
31. An old male with intestinal obstruction_____ 96
32. Cystic lesion in the pelvis of an adult female_____ 99
33. Back pain after a trauma _____ 102
34. An old male with prostate enlargment and back pain_____ 105
35. An old man with chronic back pain _____ 108
36. An old femlae with lower back pain and stiffness _____ 111
Index _____ 115

PREFACE

Since its invention in the seventies, Computerized Tomography (CT) uses and applications has grown and increased rapidly and it has become an indispensable tool in the radiology departments all over the world. It has become the first investigation of choice for multiple conditions such as strokes and head traumas. That caused CT Scanning to constitute a large portion of modern radiology departments' workload.

When we introduce medical students, interns and new Senior House Officers (SHO) to interpreting the most common findings we encounter in our daily practice, we feel the need for a small reference the contains the most common findings seen in our department within the context of the most common presentations for the patients who have these findings. That is what motivated us to write this book. Our goal is to create a simple tool to assist us in introducing CT to newcomers and to make this tool available for anyone else who is looking for a short and a simple introduction.

To prepare this book, we went over the cases we have, and chose the most illustrative ones to include them. After that, we removed any personal details that are related to our patients to maintain their privacy. Then we constructed short clinical scenarios for the cases.

Each case in this book is followed by few questions about the description of the finding(s) in the CT scan, the differential diagnoses or the diagnosis of the case condition and about the conditions themselves. These questions are answered briefly in the answers and discussion part to give the reader a simple idea about the findings and diseases.

We tried to vary the cases we chose to include in this book to cover the widest possible range of conditions and regions. You will be able to find noncontrast enhanced CT and contrast-enhanced CT scans of many regions like brain, paranasal sinuses, temporal bone, chest, abdomen, pelvis, and spine.

Your feedback is always welcomed and appreciated. If you have any suggestions to improve this book or for cases to be included in the next edition, then please send these to us on this email address:

abdallamutwakilgamal@gmail.com

We are looking forward to receiving your comments and feedback, so we can use them to improve this book in the next editions.

Mahmoud H. Milad

Abdalla M. Gamal

1. ACUTE LIMBS WEAKNESS AND INABILITY TO SPEAK

A 69-year-old male with acute weakness of the left side of his face, his left arm and left leg was brought to hospital. His initial CT scan was normal. The image below is taken from a head CT scan that he had 3 days later.

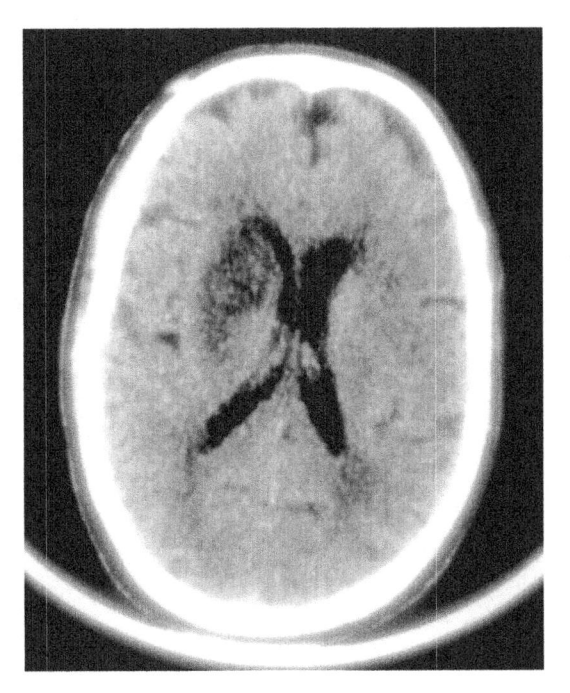

Questions

1. What is the finding seen in this scan?

2. What is the diagnosis?

Answers and Discussion

The image shows a hypodense lesion in the territory of the left middle cerebral artery at the region of the right basal ganglia and internal capsule. The lesion has a mass effect in the form of mild compression of the right lateral ventricle. These findings are consistent with an acute infarction in the Lenticulostriate arteries on the right side.

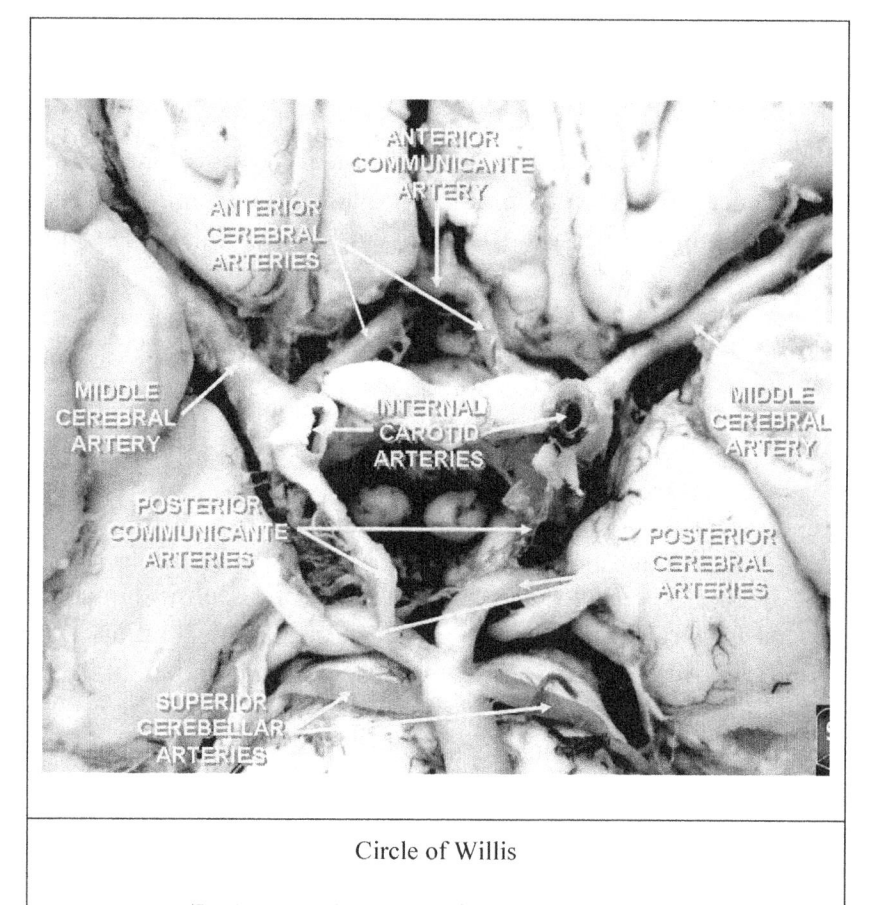

Circle of Willis

(By Anatomist90. Licensed under CC BY-SA 3.0)

The middle cerebral artery is a branch of the internal carotid artery, and it has four parts (M1, M2, M3 and M4). M1 is called the spheniodal branch and it is the segment that extends from the origin of the artery to its bifurcation. This segment has four branches; some of them (lateral lenticulostriate arteries) supply the putamen, external capsule, and a part of the internal capsule. The remaining part of the blood supply of the basal ganglia and internal capsule comes from the anterior cerebral artery branches. Medial lenticulostriate arteries, which arise from A1 segment of the anterior cerebral artery, supply the caudate nucleus and the anterior limb of the internal capsule. The recurrent artery of Heubner, a branch of A2 segment of the anterior cerebral artery, supplies the internal capsule.

Infarcts in the middle cerebral artery territory are common. They usually present with motor symptoms (hemiparesis), sensory symptoms (hemisensory loss), visual symptoms (hemianopia) and the patient may have aphasia.

Ischemic strokes have three main phases and each of these phases differ from the others on CT scan:

- Hyperacute phase (0-6 hours)
- Acute phase (6-24 hours)
- Subacute phase (1-7 days)

In the hyperacute phase, no signs can be seen in noncontrast enhanced CT scan apart from hyperdense middle cerebral artery and obscured lentiform nucleus in some cases of middle cerebral artery occlusion. In general, changes start to appear in the acute stage. These changes include effacement of sulci and loss of grey-white matter differentiation (both of which are cause by edema), in addition to hypodense basal ganglia and insula ribbon sign. Insula ribbon sign is the decrease of the density of insular cortex due to ischemia in some cases of middle cerebral artery occlusion. Changes seen in subacute infarcts include hypodense areas, hemorrhagic transformation and compression of CSF spaces (ventricles, cisterns) with or without midline shift.

2. ACUTE LEFT SIDED WEAKNESS

A 57-year-old male had an acute weakness of his left upper and lower limbs. He is a known case of Hypertension on and off treatment. On admission, his blood pressure was 240/120 mm Hg and he had left sided hemiparesis and sensory loss. The image below is taken from his head CT scan.

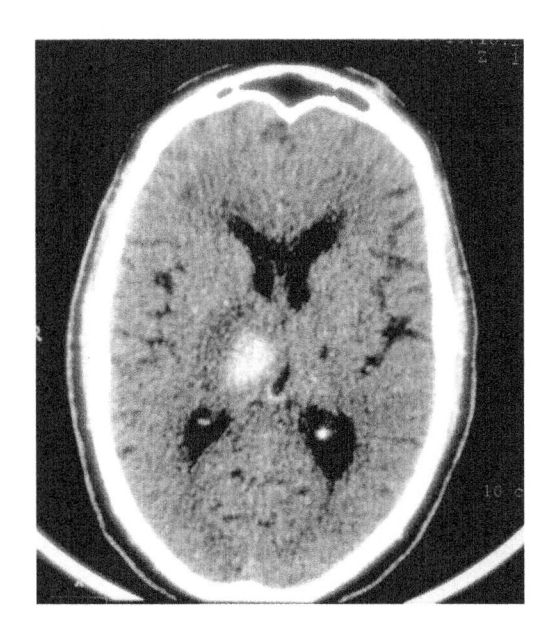

Questions

1. What does the CT image show?

2. What is the likely diagnosis?

Answers and Discussion

The image shows a hyperdense lesion in the region of the right thalamus. The lesion is surrounded by a hypodense rim and is compressing the right lateral ventricle and is causing a mild shift of the midline to the left side. The most likely diagnosis is intracerebral hemorrhage.

Cerebrovascular accident (CVA) or Stroke is a condition in which there is a reduction or complete obstruction of blood flow to a specific area in the brain and that can lead to brain cell death and permanent disability. There are two types of strokes: ischemic and hemorrhagic. Hemorrhagic strokes are less common than the ischemic ones and they constitute about 20% of all strokes.

Hemorrhagic strokes can be classified according to the site of bleeding into intracerebral hemorrhages and subarachnoid hemorrhages. The most common cause for hemorrhagic strokes is high blood pressure. There are some other less common causes such as coagulopathies, thrombolytic therapy, anticoagulant therapy, vasculitis, aneurysms, and arteriovenous malformations.

The presentation of the patient depends on the affected area and can include symptoms like confusion, weakness of limbs, loss of the ability to speak, convulsions or headache. On examination some of the following signs might be found: hemiparesis, loss of sensation, aphasia, hemianopia, confusion, facial weakness, or apraxia.

The appearance of the hemorrhage on noncontrast enhanced CT scan of brain depends on the age of the hemorrhage:

- Acute hemorrhage (less than 1 week old):
    - Appears as a hyperdense area (density between 50 and 70 HU).
    - If the patient has low hemoglobin or a bleeding disorder, it might appear as an isodense area.

- Subacute hemorrhage (1-6 weeks old):
  - Appear as an isodense area.
- Chronic hemorrhage (older than 6 weeks old):
  - Appears as a hypodense area.
  - If there is a rebleeding, then the areas of rebleeding will appear as small hyperdense areas inside the hypodense old hemorrhage.

The mortality rate of patients with hemorrhagic strokes is very high. Only 40% of patients live longer than one year after having a hemorrhagic stroke.

3. AN OLD FEMALE WITH LOSS OF CONCIOUSNESS

A 79-year-old female was brought unconscious to the emergency department. A CT scan of head without contrast was requested to rule out intracranial pathologies. The images below are taken from her head CT scan.

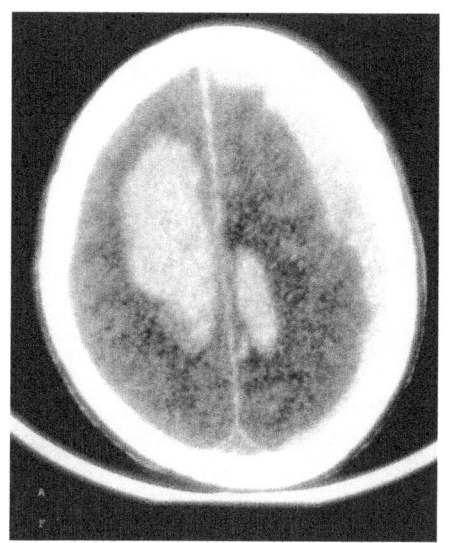

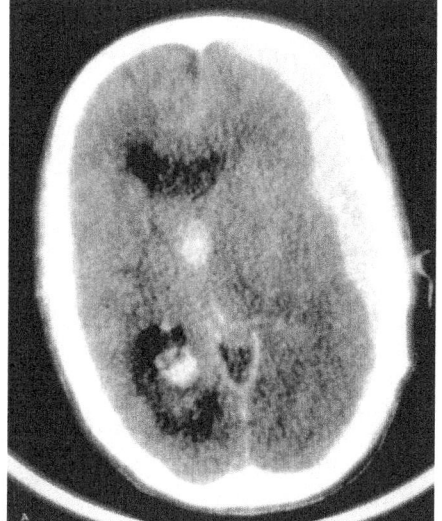

Questions

1. What are the findings seen in the patient CT scan?

2. What is the diagnosis?

3. What are the types of intracranial hemorrhages and what are their most common causes?

Answers and Discussion

The images show hyperdense crescent-shaped extraaxial collection in the left frontoparietal region with shift of the midline to the left side and hyperdense ventricles. These findings are consistent with left sided subdural hemorrhage in the left frontoparietal region and bilateral intraventricular hemorrhage inside both lateral ventricles.

Intracranial hemorrhages can be classified into:

- Intraaxial hemorrhages:
    o Intraparenchymal hemorrhage
    o Intraventricular hemorrhage
- Extraaxial hemorrhages:
    o Epidural hemorrhage
    o Subdural hemorrhage
    o Subarachnoid hemorrhage

Classification of intracranial hemorrhage into intra- and extraaxial hemorrhage depends on the location of the hemorrhage. Intraaxial hemorrhages are inside the brain while extraaxial hemorrhages are outside the brain. Intraaxial hemorrhages are usually the more dangerous ones.

In this case, we see one type of extraaxial hemorrhage (subdural hemorrhage) and one type of intraaxial hemorrhage (intraventricular hemorrhage). Each of these types can occur alone or with other types and intracranial pathologies.

In subdural hemorrhage, blood accumulates between the brain and the dura. It has many causes, the most common of them are: trauma and anticoagulant therapy. Very young people, very old people and alcoholics are at more risk of having this type of hemorrhage. Subdural hemorrhages can be acute or chronic and can have sudden onset. They can present with loss of consciousness or they can develop slowly and cause headache, vomiting, confusion, hemiparesis, or convulsions.

The appearance of subdural hemorrhage on CT scan depends on the age of the hemorrhage. In all times, it will appear as a crescent shaped lesion between the brain and the skull. In acute phase, it will appear hyperdense. In subacute phase, it will be isodense and in the chronic phase, it will have hypodense appearance.

Intraventricular hemorrhage can be primary (involving only the ventricles) or secondary (extending to ventricles from other location). Usual causes of primary intraventricular hemorrhages are trauma, tumours, aneurysms, and AVM in choroid plexus. Secondary intraventricular hemorrhage can be caused by extension of intraparenchymal or subarachnoid hemorrhage to the ventricles. Usually, there are focal neurological signs with primary intraventricular hemorrhage, and the symptoms tend to be general. Symptoms include sudden headache, vomiting, or change in consciousness level. Mortality rate in patients with intraventricular hemorrhage is about 50-80%.

4. CHRONIC HEADACHE AND VOMITING

A 44-year-old female complains of chronic headache that started few months ago and is associated with early morning vomiting. The images below are taken from her contrast-enhanced CT scan of head.

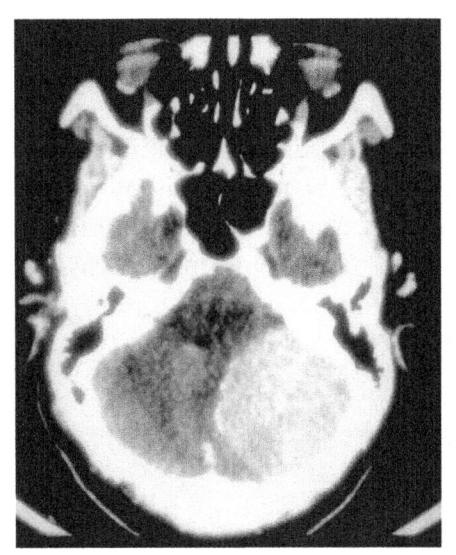

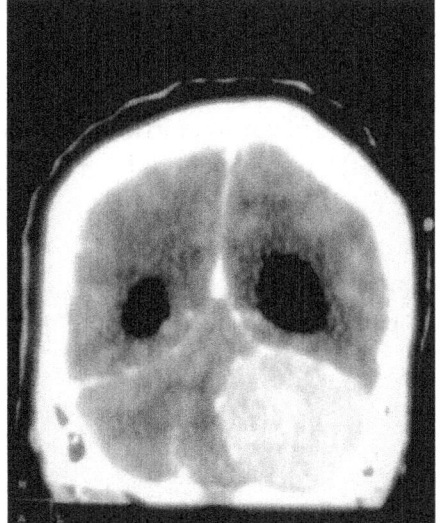

Questions

1. What does the CT Images show?

2. What is the most likely diagnosis?

3. What are the other symptoms that can be caused by this lesion?

Answers and Discussion

The CT images show a single well-defined extraaxial infratentorial focal lesion in the left side of the posterior cranial fossa with intense homogeneous enhancement. The lesion compresses the left cerebellar hemisphere and causes a shift of the midline to the left side with compression of the 4th ventricle. The most likely diagnosis is meningioma.

Meningiomas are brain or spinal cord tumours that arise from the meninges. They are usually benign and they constitute about 20% of all primary brain tumours. The presentation of meningiomas depends on their site and size. When they are in the posterior cranial fossa, they can present in many different ways in addition to presenting with headache and vomiting. The most common of these additional presentations are: cranial nerve dysfunction, vermian syndrome, ataxia (truncal or limb), nystagmus, and dysmetria.

Other tumours can arise in the location of this lesion (in the posterior cranial fossa). These tumours are intraaxial tumours and they constitute about 15-20% of all brain tumours in adults. These tumours include:

- Metastases
- Haemangioblastoma
- Astrocytomas
- Medulloblastomas

Cerebellar metastases are the most common type of posterior cranial fossa tumours. The most common sources for these metastases are lung and breast cancers. Haemangioblastomas are benign tumours that arise from the central nervous system vessels. They are the most common primary tumours in the cerebellum, and they constitute about 7-10% of the posterior fossa tumours seen in adults. Astrocytomas and medulloblastomas are rare in adults.

The differentiation between extra- and intraaxial tumours depends on finding some characteristics that identifies the extraaxial location of the tumour like:

- Having wide dural base
- CSF cleft sign
- Finding cortical grey matter between the lesion and the white matter.

5. AN ADULT MALE WITH CONVLSIONS

A 27-year-old male with recurrent convulsions was admitted to the department of medicine. The patient is a known case of small cell lung carcinoma. His temperature was normal and his white cells count was 8,000. The images below are taken from his head CT scan before and after contrast administration.

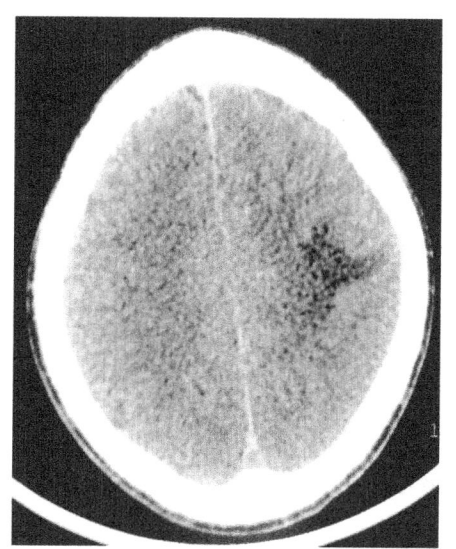

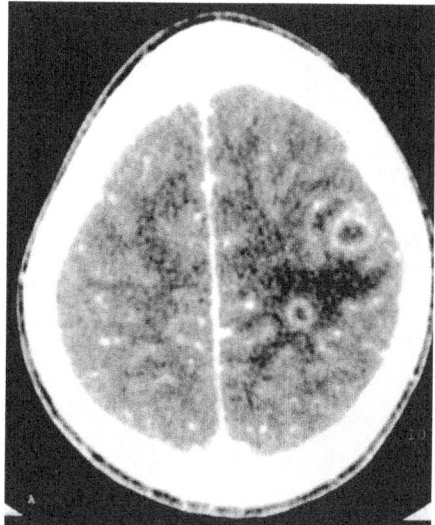

Questions

1. What are the findings seen in this scan?

2. What is the differential diagnosis for these findings?

3. What is the most likely diagnosis?

Answers and Discussion

The CT images show an ill-defined hypodense area in the upper part of the left parietal lobe with finger-like projections before the administration of contrast. After contrast administration, two well-defined spheroid hypodense lesions with ring enhancement are seen. The two lesions are surrounded by perifocal edema.

The differential diagnosis of brain lesions with ring enhancement on CT scan includes:

- CNS Infections:
    o Brain abscess
    o Tuberculoma
    o Neurocysticercosis
- CNS tumours:
    o Metastasis
    o Glioblastoma multiforme
- In HIV positive patients:
    o CNS toxoplasmosis
    o CNS lymphoma

The most likely diagnosis in this case is cerebral metastasis from the patient's lung carcinoma.

The most common sources of metastasis to the brain are lung tumours, breast tumours, gastrointestinal tumours, and genitourinary tumours. Metastatic tumours represent about third of the tumours found in the brain.

Some patients with brain metastasis are asymptomatic, but the majority has one or more of the following symptoms: headache, vomiting, convulsions, focal neurological deficit, or ataxia.

Up to 40% of patients with malignancies have brain metastasis on the time of diagnosis, and those metastasis can be detected using various imaging modalities. The majority of those metastases are found in cerebrum (about 80%). Although brain metastases are thought to be usually multiple, studies show that about half of the patients with brain metastasis have solitary metastasis. Metastatic tutumours in brain can have any density (hypo-, iso- or hyperdense), and any types of enhancement. The usual finding with different types of metastasis is the surrounding brain edema.

Although contrast-enhanced CT scan is very sensitive in detecting brain metastases, MRI with contrast is considered the best choice for looking for metastasis in the brain. The reason behind this is that contrast-enhanced CT scan misses some small metastasis especially if they are adjacent to skull bones.

6. AN OLD MALE WITH RIGHT SIDED FACIAL PALSY

An old male with weight loss and right sided facial palsy was referred to the radiology department for a CT scan. The images below are taken from his head CT scan before and after contrast administration.

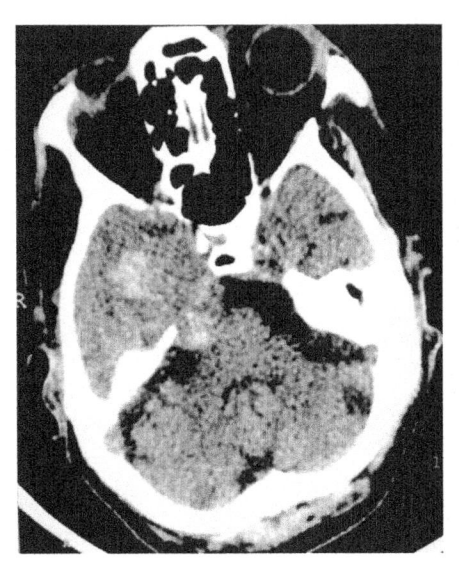

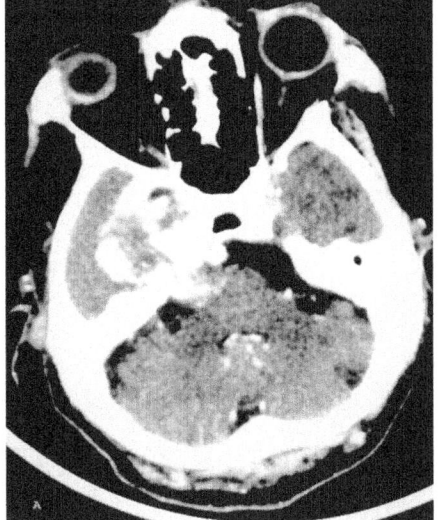

Questions

1. What is the finding seen in this scan?

2. What is the differential diagnosis of this finding?

3. What are the causes of this condition?

Answers and Discussion

Before administration of contrast, an ill-defined heterogeneous focal lesion is seen in the right temporal lobe with extension to the posterior cranial fossa. The mass contains hyperdense areas that can be hemorrhage or calcification. After contrast administration, the lesion has strong heterogonous enhancement.

Differential diagnosis for this lesion includes the differential diagnoses of supratentorial intraaxial masses with heterogeneous enhancement. The most common of these masses are:

- Oligodendroglioma
- Gliosarcoma
- Metastatic deposits

Oligodendroglioma is a slow growing brain tumor that usually occurs in middle aged patients. It is characterized by its heterogeneous appearance on noncontrast enhanced CT scan with calcification seen in up to 90% of the cases and cystic degeneration in about 20% of the cases. It usually involves the cerebral cortex and subcortical areas. Most common presentations of Oligodendroglioma are convulsions, headache, and focal neurological deficits.

Gliosarcoma is a rare brain tumour that is thought to arise from the vascular components of Glioblastoma multiform. It usually presents with symptoms of raised intracranial pressure. It can cause convulsions and focal neurological deficits. On contrast-enhanced CT scan, it is characterized by its heterogeneous enhancement and its invasion of the dura. It can involve the skull bones in some cases.

Cerebral metastases are usually iso- or hypodense lesions found at the grey-white matter interface. They can be surrounded by various degrees of brain edema. And sometimes there is no brain edema around them. Spontaneous hemorrhage can occur inside those metastases any time. These tumours represent about half of all brain tumours. The most common tumours that metastasize to the brain are lung, breast, and gastrointestinal tract tumours.

7. AN INCIDENTAL INTRACRANIAL CYST FOUND ON HEAD CT

The images below show an incidental finding on head CT scan that was done for a 55-year-old male.

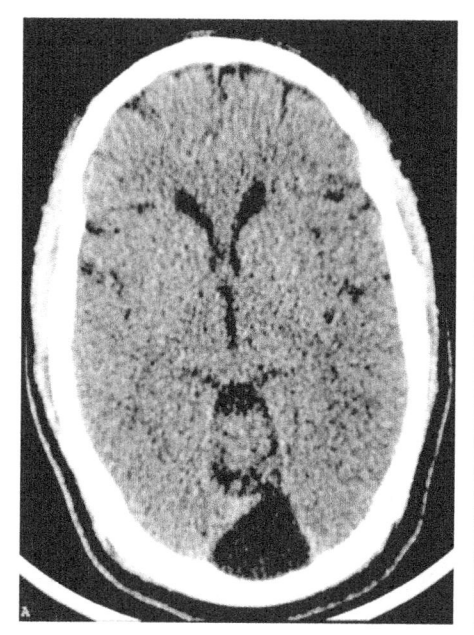

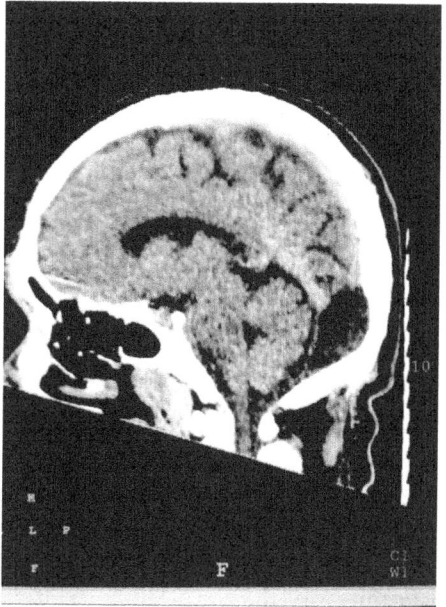

Questions

1. What is the finding seen in this scan?

2. What is the most likely diagnosis?

3. What is the differential diagnosis of this finding?

Answers and Discussion

The images show a well-defined extraaxial cystic lesion in the posterior cranial fossa behind the cerebellum. The most likely diagnosis is subarachnoid cyst.

A large number of the intracranial pathologies might have a cystic component. But the Differential diagnosis of pure intracranial cyst includes:

- Subarachnoid cyst
- Hydatid cyst
- Dermoid cyst
- Epidermoid cyst

All of the cysts mentioned above have no enhancement on contrast administration. Differentiation between those cysts can be difficult based on CT scan alone, but each of them has some features that might help in reaching a diagnosis from the CT scan.

First of all, hydatid cyst is the only intraaxial cyst from the list above. All other cysts are extraaxial. Dermoid cysts are usually found near the midline and have fat-density contents. Epidermoid cysts can be lobulated and are usually found in the posterior cranial fossa (less commonly they are found in the middle cranial fossa or parasellar region). Subarachnoid cysts are usually found in the middle cranial fossa, but can be found in multiple other locations like the posterior cranial fossa.

Subarachnoid cysts are benign intracranial cystic lesions that occur due to failure of the fusion of meninges. They contain CSF and their size is variable. There most common sites are middle cranial fossa, cerebellopontine angle, and suprasellar area. They are usually asymptomatic and are found in up to 1% of the general population.

Hydatid cysts are caused by Echinococcus granulosus, Echinococcus multilocularis or Echinococcus alveolaris. Intracranial cyst formation occurs in about 2% of patient with hydatid disease. The patients usually present with symptoms of raised intracranial pressure (like headache and convulsions).

Dermoid cysts are rare congenital cysts that are thought to result from the entrapment of the surface epithelium in the lines of fusion. They commonly present in the 4th to 6th decade of life because of their slow growth. The most common presentations of patients with dermoid cysts are headache and convulsions.

Epidermoid cysts can be congenital or acquired. When they are congenital, they arise from entrapment of ectodermal cells. Acquired epidermoid cysts arise due to trauma. Intracranial epidermoid cysts are usually congenital. Their most common presentations are headache and cranial nerve palsy (especially of trigeminal, facial or vestibule-cochlear nerves).

8. AN INFANT WITH LARGE HEAD

After recovering form meningitis, a 6-month-old boy suffered from gradual increase in his head size. On examination, he had a large head with a head circumference that is above the 95th centile for his age and a tense bulging anterior fontanel. The images below are taken from his noncontrast enhanced CT scan.

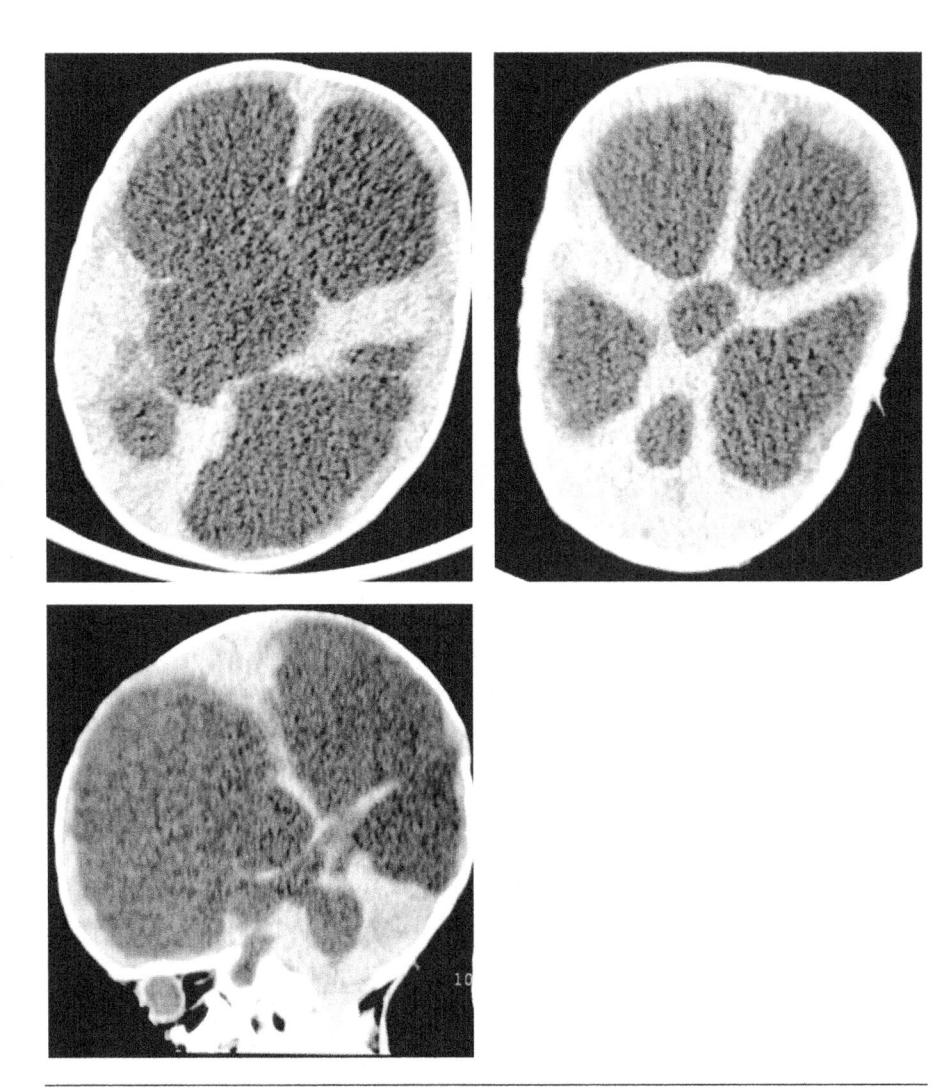

Questions

1. What are the findings seen in this scan?

2. What is the diagnosis?

3. What are the causes of this condition?

Answers and Discussion

There is severe dilatation in both lateral, 3rd and 4th ventricles in this patient CT scan images with dilatation of the quadrigeminal cistern. These findings are consistent with communicating hydrocephalus.

Hydrocephalus is the dilatation of the ventricular system due to CSF overproduction or decreased CSF absorption. According to its mechanism, it can be classified into non-obstructive hydrocephalus (in which there is increased production of CSF by choroid plexuses and obstructive hydrocephalus (in which there is decreased absorption of CSF due to obstruction).

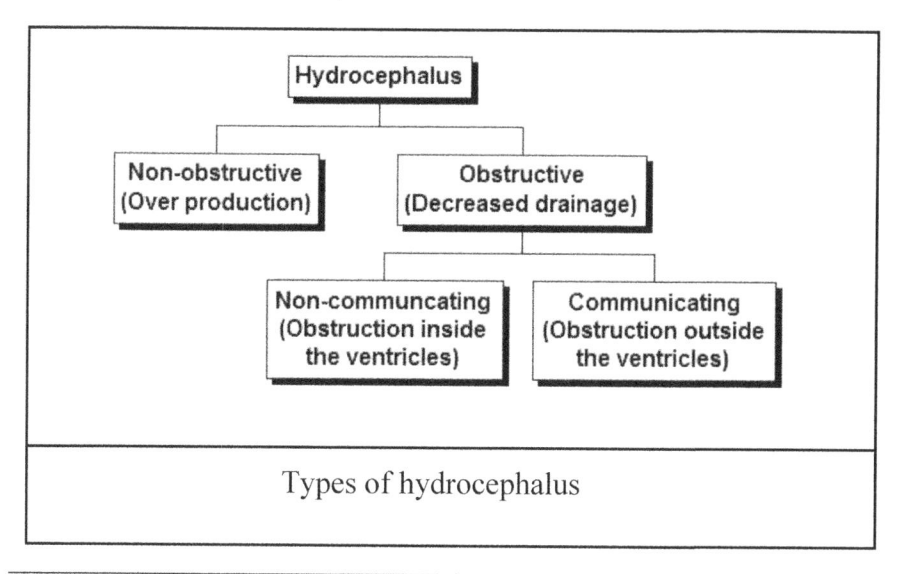

```
                    ┌──────────────┐
                    │ Hydrocephalus │
                    └──────┬───────┘
              ┌────────────┴────────────┐
   ┌──────────────────┐         ┌──────────────────┐
   │  Non-obstructive │         │    Obstructive   │
   │ (Over production)│         │(Decreased drainage)│
   └──────────────────┘         └────────┬─────────┘
                              ┌──────────┴──────────┐
                   ┌──────────────────┐   ┌──────────────────┐
                   │  Non-communcating│   │   Communicating  │
                   │(Obstruction inside)│  │(Obstruction outside)│
                   │   the ventricles │   │   the ventricles │
                   └──────────────────┘   └──────────────────┘
```

Types of hydrocephalus

Simple common cases in CT scan

The site of the obstruction is used to classify obstructive hydrocephalus further into non-communicating type (in which there is obstruction inside the ventricular system) and communicating type (in which there is obstruction outside the ventricular system, at the arachnoid villi).

The earliest signs of hydrocephalus include dilation of the temporal horns of lateral ventricles and dilated oval 3rd ventricle. CT scan can also show effacement of brain sulci, rounded frontal and occipital horns of lateral ventricles. The diameter of the normal frontal horn of lateral ventricle in people younger than 40 years of age is less than 12mm and in people older than 40 years of age is less than 15mm. the width of the 3rd ventricle in less than 5mm in children and less than 7-9mm in adults.

The presentation of patients with hydrocephalus depends on their age. In infants, where the skull sutures are still open, the presentation is usually a progressively enlarging head with bulging anterior fontanel, vomiting, or change in the level of consciousness.

The most common causes of acquired communicating hydrocephalus are:

- Postinfectious.
- Posthemorrhagic.
- CNS tumours.

9. A TEENAGE FEMALE WITH HYDROCEPHALUS AND SHUNT

A 14-year-old female with congenital hydrocephalus had a shunt inserted to drain the CSF when she was an infant. She had a brain CT scan to assess the shunt function. The images below are taken from her scan.

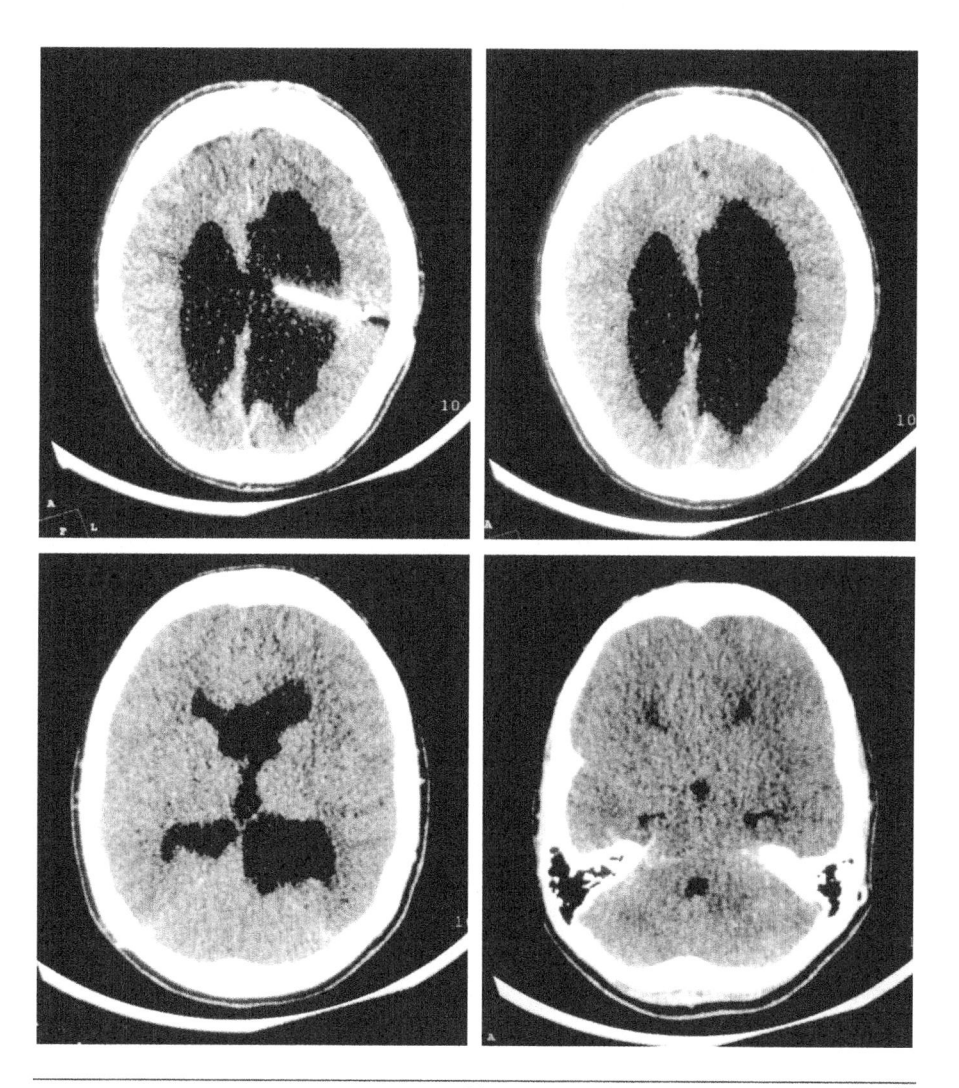

Questions

1. What type of hydrocephalus does this girl have?

2. What are the most common causes of this type?

3. What are the most common complications of ventriculoperitoneal shunts?

Answers and Discussion

This girl has non-communicating obstructive hydrocephalus with dilatation in both lateral ventricles and 3rd ventricle and a normal 4th ventricle. The most likely site of obstruction is at the aqueduct of Sylvius. Non-communicating hydrocephalus has multiple causes. The most common of these causes are:

- Agenesis of the foramen of Monro.
- Aqueductal stenosis
- Malformations:
    - Chiari malformation
    - Dandy-Walker malformation
- Tumour
- Abscess
- Intraventricular hematomas.

Some of these causes are congenital (for example, aqueduct stenosis, Chiari malformation, and Dandy-Walker malformations) and some are acquired (such as tumours, hematomas and abscesses). From the case history, her problem is congenital. The CT scan images show a normal posterior cranial fossa, and that excludes both Chiari malformation and Dandy-Walker malformations. The most likely cause for hydrocephalus in this case is congenital aqueduct stenosis.

Ventriculoperitoneal shunts have many complications. These complications include:

- Shunt obstruction.
- Shunt infection.
- Overdrainage.
- Subdural hematoma.
- Abdominal complications (such as bowel perforation, hernias, and pseudocyst formation).

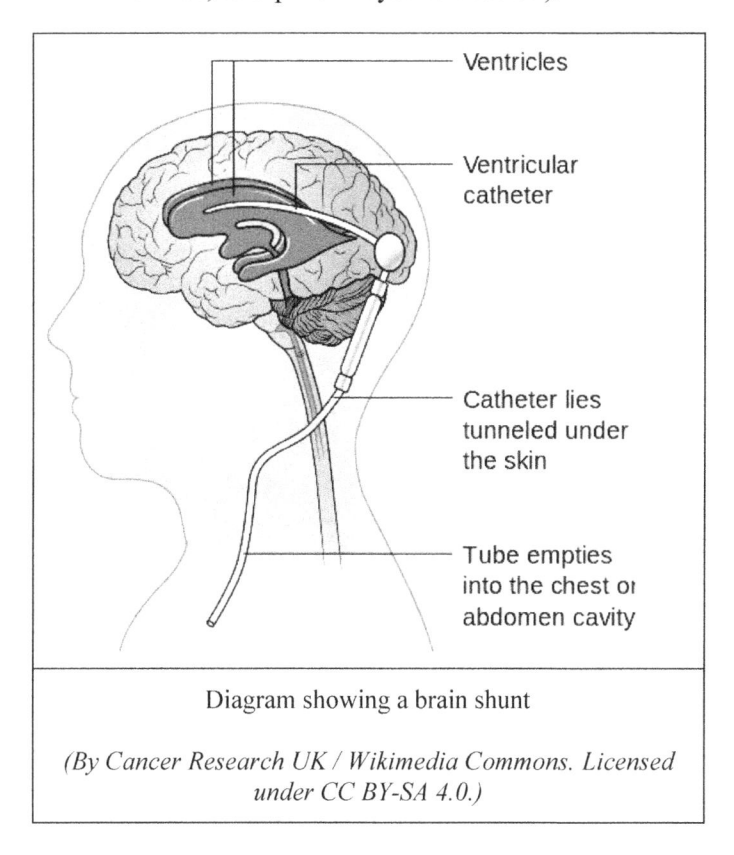

Diagram showing a brain shunt

(By Cancer Research UK / Wikimedia Commons. Licensed under CC BY-SA 4.0.)

10. HYPERDENSE SULCI AFTER A HEAD TRAUMA.

A 26-year-old male who had a head trauma was sent to the radiology department for head CT scan. Image below are taken from his head CT scan.

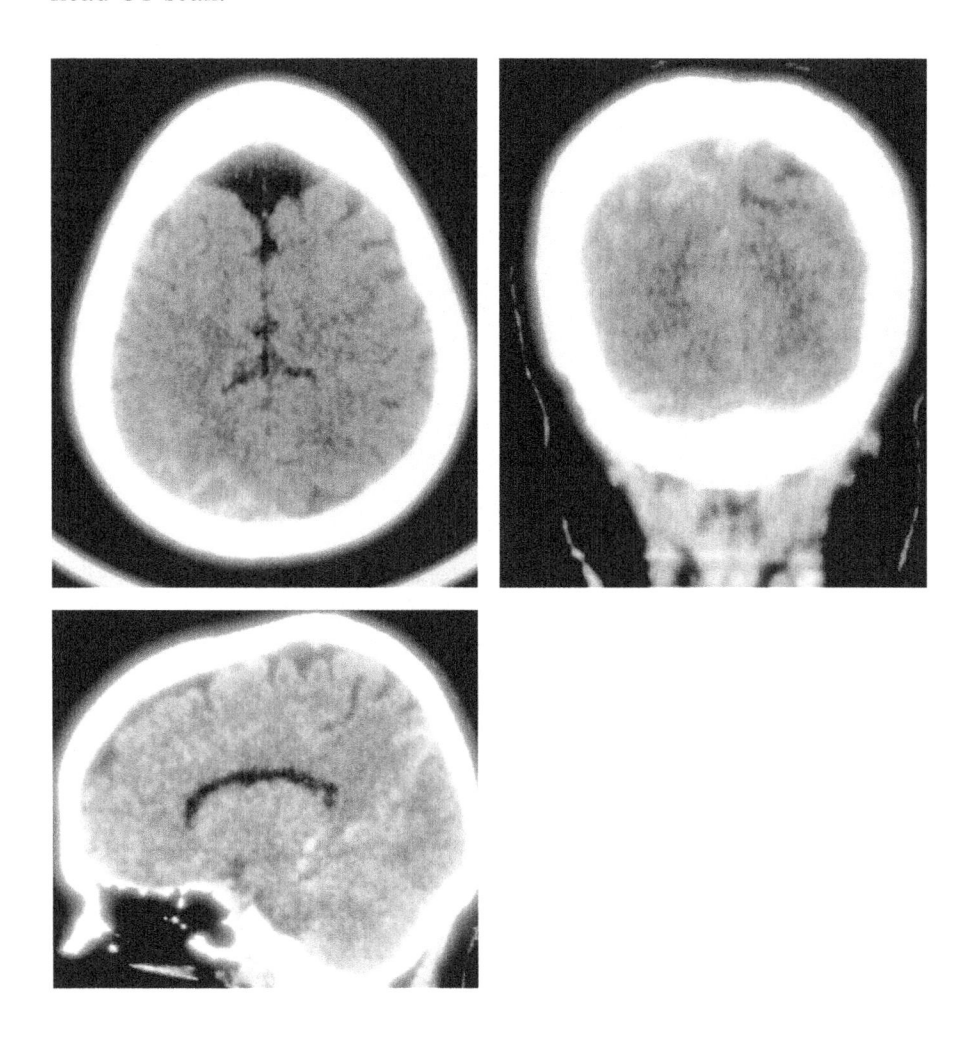

Questions

1. What are the findings seen in this scan?

2. What is the diagnosis?

3. What are the causes of this condition?

Answers and Discussion

The CT images show hyperdense sulci in the posterior part of the right parietal lobe and in the right occipital lobe. This is consistent with subarachnoid hemorrhage.

Subarachnoid hemorrhage has many causes. It can traumatic as we have seen in this case, or it can be spontaneous. Spontaneous subarachnoid hemorrhage is caused by ruptured berry aneurysm in most of cases, but it can be caused by arteriovenous malformation, pituitary apoplexy, cocaine abuse, or anticoagulant therapy.

The classical presentation of subarachnoid hemorrhage is thunderclap headache which is a sudden, diffuse and severe headache that can last for few seconds or up to two weeks. This headache can be associated with neck pain, vomiting, transient loss of consciousness or convulsions.

Differential diagnosis of findings that suggest subarachnoid hemorrhage on CT scan includes:

- Subarachnoid hemorrhage
- Pseudo-subarachnoid hemorrhage
    - Meningitis (Bacterial meningitis and Tuberculous meningitis).

- Significant hypoxic-ischemic injury (for example, in patients with post-resuscitation anoxic encephalopathy)
- Spontaneous intracranial hypotension).

There are many scales for grading subarachnoid hemorrhage such as Hunt and Hess scale, Botterell et al. scale, The World Federation of Neurological Surgeons Scale (WFNS) and Fisher Scale. Each one of these scales has different advantages and disadvantages. The Fisher scale is simple and depends only on the initial findings on the CT scan that was done on admission. The following table shows the different grades of this scale.

\multicolumn{2}{c}{The Fisher scale for grading subarachnoid hemorrhage}	
Grade	Description
Grade 1	No blood visualized on CT scan
Grade 2	CT scan shows A diffuse deposition or thin layer with all vertical layers of blood (interhemispheric fissure, insular cistern, ambient cistern) less than 1 mm thick
Grade 3	Localized clots and/or vertical layers of blood 1 mm or greater in thickness seen in CT scan
Grade 4	CT scan shows Diffuse or no subarachnoid blood, but with intracerebral or intraventricular clots

11. A DROWZY CHILD AFTER HEAD TRAUMA

A 3-year-old female with drowsiness after head trauma underwent CT scan of head. The images below are taken from her noncontrast enhanced CT scan of head.

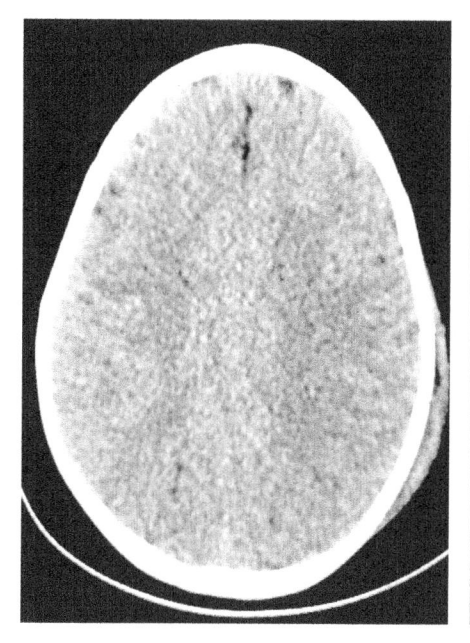

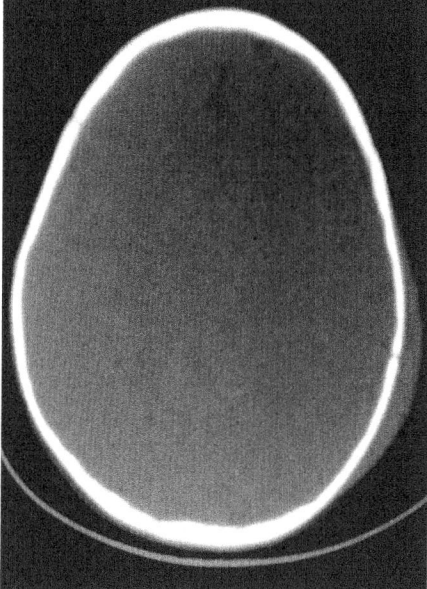

Questions

1. What are the findings seen in this scan?

2. What are the indications for head CT in cases of head trauma?

Answers and Discussion

The CT scan images show hazy brain parenchyma with flattening of sulci and gyri. In addition to this, there is a linear fracture in the right occipital bone and a hematoma in the scalp overlying the fracture. These findings are consistent with brain edema, linear skull fracture and scalp hematoma.

There are many indications for CT scan of head in patients with head trauma. These indications include:

- Suspected skull fractures (open, depressed, or skull base fractures).
- Focal neurological deficit, convulsions, or vomiting more than one time after the trauma.
- Abnormal level of consciousness (Glasgow coma scale below 13 at admission or below 15 two hours after admission).

There are three types of skull fractures: linear, depressed and skull base fractures. Skull fractures can be also classified according to the state of skin and soft tissues above them into open fractures (associated with skin and soft tissues injuries and are exposed to external environment) and closed fractures (with intact skin and soft tissues over them). These fractures can occur with a normal brain below them or they can result in intracranial hemorrhage and/or brain edema. CT scan is the best method to visualize these fractures and it is replacing x-ray in this task quickly.

Linear skull fractures are the most common type of skull fractures seen in trauma cases. These fractures are usually uncomplicated, but they can be dangerous if they occur in the location of intracranial blood vessels. Most patients with this type of fractures are asymptomatic.

Depressed skull fractures are comminuted fractures that result from blunt trauma to head. In this type of fractures, the fragments are displaced downwards which causes a high risk of brain injury. Patients with this type of fractures might lose consciousness or remain conscious. The presentation also depends on the associated injuries.

Skull base fractures represent about fifth of all skull fractures. They can occur in the anterior cranial fossa or middle cranial fossa. Their presentation depends on their site. These fractures can cause tears in the meninges and that leads to the CSF leakage associated with them and increases the risk of having meningitis in patients with these fractures.

Clues to the presence of skull base fractures	
Type of fracture	**Possible signs**
Anterior cranial fossa fracture	• Periorbital ecchymosis • Subconjunctival hemorrhage • Bleeding from nose • CSF leakage from nose
Middle cranial fossa fracture	• Bruising over ear or mastoid process • Bleeding from ear • CSF leakage from ear
Both fractures can cause injury of cranial nerves.	

If skull fractures are not complicated and the patient has no brain edema or hemorrhage, then he might need no treatment or he might only need admission for observation. If there is contamination of open skull fracture, then antibiotics might be used. Some depressed skull fractures might require surgical intervention.

12. AN ADULT MALE WITH FACIAL TRAUMA

A 23-year-old male with motor vehicle accident and head trauma was sent for CT scan of brain and facial bones. The images below are taken from his scan.

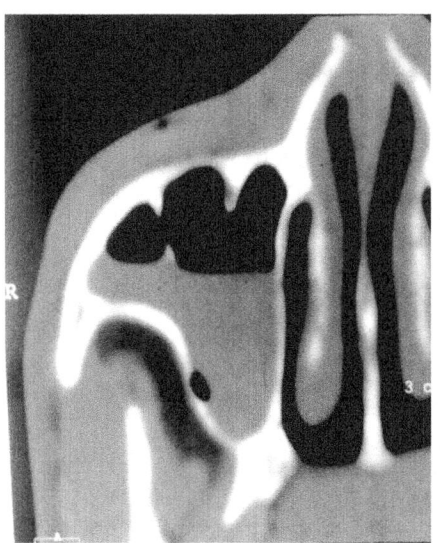

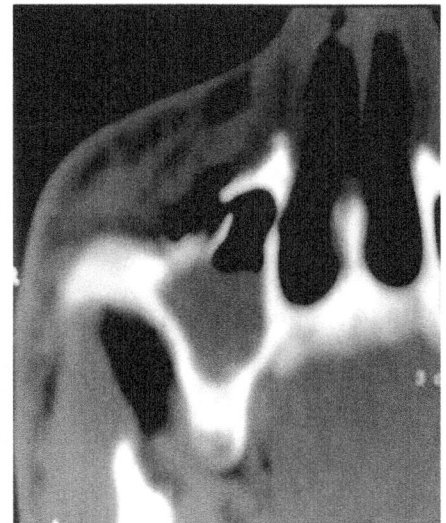

Questions

1. What are the findings seen in this scan?

2. What is the diagnosis?

Answers and Discussion

The images show fracture in the anterior wall of the right maxillary sinus with partially opaque right maxillary sinus. These findings are consistent with a zygomatico-maxillary fracture with hemosinus.

Facial injuries have multiple causes. They can result from motor vehicle accidents, assaults, falls, sport injuries, gunshots, and blasts injuries. Structures affected by facial injuries can include soft tissues (with injuries such as brusies, lacerations, and abrasions) and/or bones with variable fractures such as nasal bone fractures, maxillary or mandibular fractures. The seriousness of facial injuries is caused by the associated injures to brain or eyes or the obstruction of airways that can occur with them. In addition to this, sometimes the severe bleeding associated with these injuries can be fatal.

Suspicion of a maxillofacial fracture after facial trauma is raised when any of the following features is found on examination of the face:

- Asymmtry of the two halves of the face
- Nasal deviation or depression
- Pupils are not at the same level
- Flat cheecks
- Subconjuncival hemorrhage

The most common fracture that results from a facial trauma is fracture of the nose. This fracture can be diagnosed easily from the clinical examination and skull x-ray. If other fractures are suspeced, then an CT scan of facial bones is necessary.

There are three special types of facial fractures that were described by a french surgeon called René Le Fort. These fractures are called Le Fort fractures and they involve pterygoid processes with combination of other fractures.

Simple common cases in CT scan

- Le Fort I fractures: are also called the floating fractures. They are caused by trauma to the lower part of maxilla. In this type of fractures, there is horizontal fracture line with separation of the alveolar process of the maxilla and palate from the upper face.
- Le Fort II fractures: also known as the pyramidal fractures. These fracture result from direct trauma to the midface. In them, the fracture line extends from the nasal bridge to the maxilla and medial aspects of both orbits. In these fractures, there is separation of the midface from the skull.
- Le Fort III fractures: in these fractures, there is separation of the entire face from the skull. The fracture line passes through nasal bone, ethmoid bones, maxilla, zygoma, and skull base.

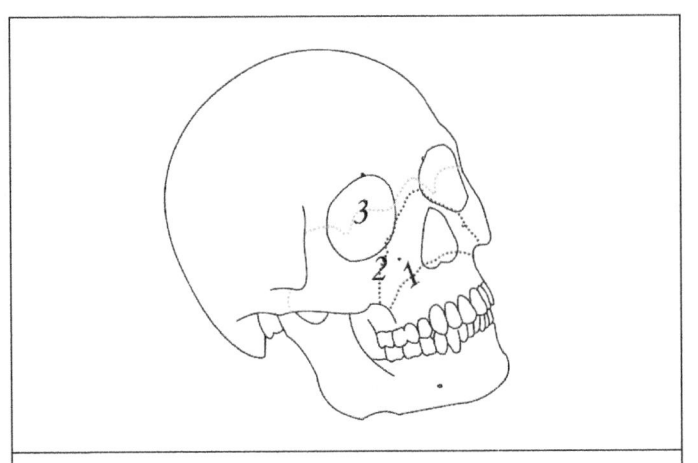

A diagram that shows Le Fort fractures. Le Fort type I (line number 1), Le Fort type II (line number 2) and Le Fort type III (line number 3).

(This diagram is a derivative of "Le Fort fractures" by RosarioVanTulpe, used under CC BY-SA 3.0. The modified diagram is licensed under CC BY-SA 3.0 by Dr Abdalla M. Gamal.)

13. AN ADULT MALE WITH A BLOW TO THE JAW

An adult male with a blow to the jaw, pain on both sides of the jaw, and restricted movements of the mandible had a CT scan to rule out fractures in the mandible. The images below are taken from his scan.

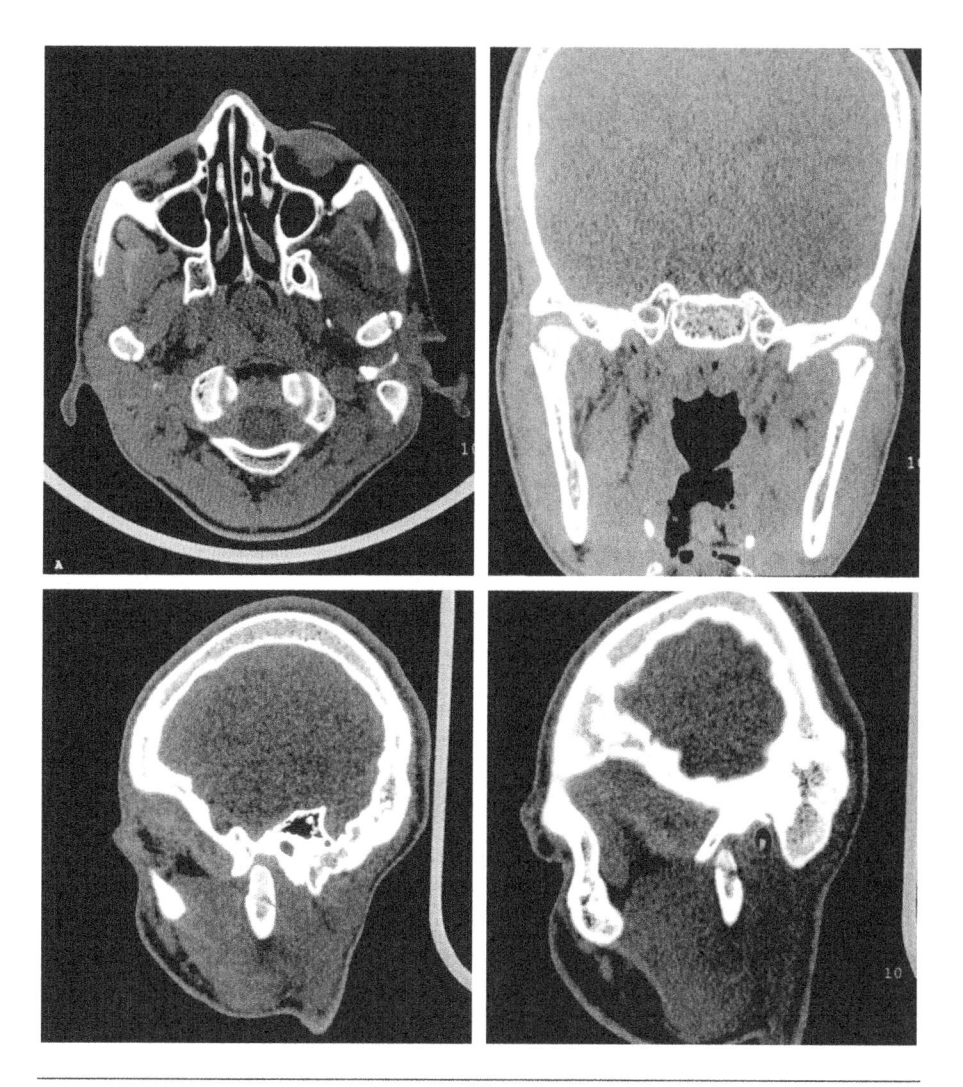

Questions

1. What are the findings seen in this scan?

2. What are the most common causes of this condition?

Answers and Discussion

The images show fractures in both condyles of the mandible with no displacement of fragments or dislocation of both temporomandibular joints.

Fractures of the mandible are the second most common facial fractures (only preceded by fractures of the nose). These fractures are usually multiple and are associated with other fractures. They can be associated with dislocation of the temporomandibular joint (TMJ).

The most common causes of mandibular fractures are motor vehicle accidents (about 40% of cases) and assaults (About 40% of cases). Other less common causes are falls, sport injuries, workplace accidents, and pathological fractures.

The pain caused by these fractures is usually aggravated by movement of the mandible. Mal-occlusion of the mouth and bruising inside the oral cavity are common findings in these fractures. On examination, the patient may also have swelling over the site of fracture or tenderness on palpation of the sites of the fractures. A gap might be palpable at site of fracture line. Care must be taken to look for other fractures because about 15% of patients with mandibular fractures have other fractures associated with them.

The most common sites of mandibular fractures are the condyles of the mandible (where about 30% of mandibular fractures occur), followed by the angle of the mandible and body of the mandible (about 25% of mandibular fractures occur at each of these sites).

The image below shows the most common sites of fractures of mandible and the frequency of fractures occurring in them.

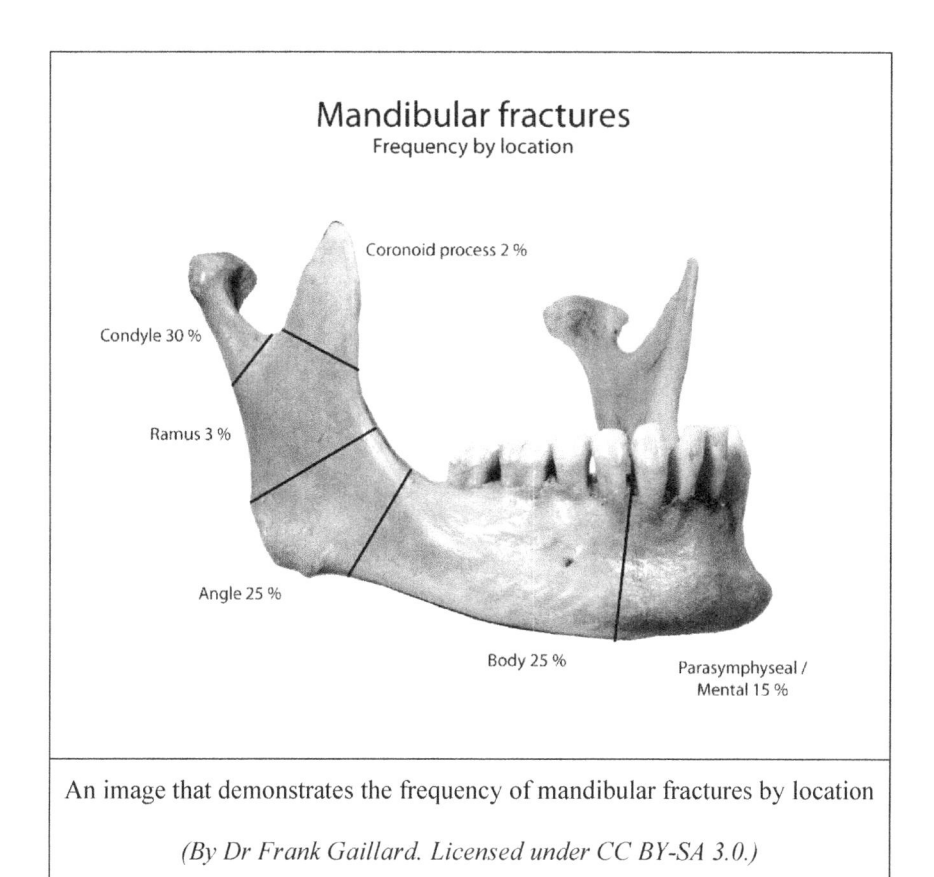

Mandibular fractures
Frequency by location

- Coronoid process 2 %
- Condyle 30 %
- Ramus 3 %
- Angle 25 %
- Body 25 %
- Parasymphyseal / Mental 15 %

An image that demonstrates the frequency of mandibular fractures by location

(By Dr Frank Gaillard. Licensed under CC BY-SA 3.0.)

Fractures of the condyles of the mandible can be unilateral or bilateral. They can present with some of the following features on examination: swelling over the temporomandibular joint on the affected side, locked mandible, laceration of the anterior wall of external auditory canal with hemorrhage from the ear on the affected side, gap over the site of the fracture, deviation of the mandible to the affected side when mouth is opened, limited mouth opening, open bite, and restricted movement of the mandible.

14. CHRONIC NASAL OBSTRUCTION AND CONGESTION

A 39-year-old female was referred from the ENT department for a noncontrast enhanced CT scan of her paranasal sinuses. She is complaining of chronic nasal obstruction and congestion. The images below are taken from her CT scan.

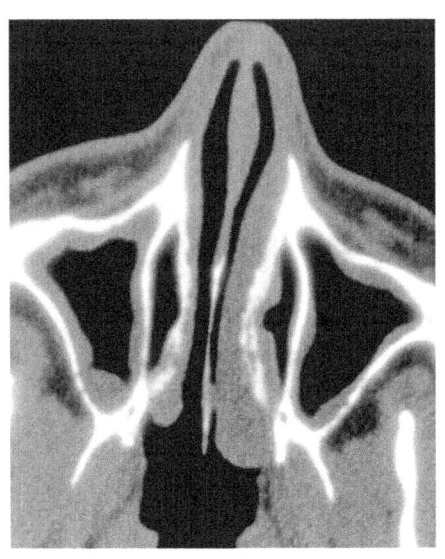

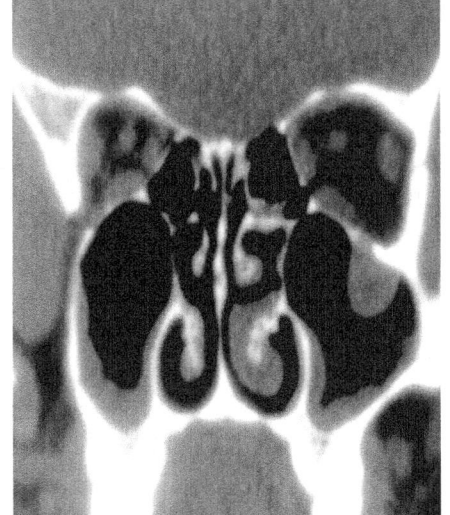

Questions

1. What are the findings seen in this scan?

2. What is the diagnosis?

3. What are the complications of this condition?

Answers and Discussion

This patient has mucosal thickening in both maxillary sinuses, a polypoidal mucosal thickening in the left maxillary sinuses and hypertrophy of the nasal conchae (mostly on the left side). These findings are consistent with chronic sinusitis with allergic rhinitis and a polyp.

Complications of chronic sinusitis include:

- In the sinuses:
  - Mucocele formation
- In orbits:
  - Preseptal cellulitis
  - Orbital cellulitis
  - Orbital abscess
- In surrounding bones:
  - Osteomyelitis
  - Subperiosteal abscess
- Intracranial complications:
  - Cavernous sinus thrombosis
  - Meningitis
  - Epidural abscess
  - Subdural abscess
  - Brain abscess

Acute and chronic sinusitis are very common conditions. They are caused by multiple organisms. The most common causes of acute sinusitis include viruses (especially rhinovirus), bacteria (Staphylococcus aureus, streptococcus pneumonia, and hemophilus influenzae) and fungi (such as Aspergillus and Curvularia). Causes of chronic sinusitis include bacteria (such as Staphylococcus aureus, streptococcus pneumonia, and hemophilus influenzae) and fungi (most commonly Aspergillus species and Cryptococcus neoformans).

Presentations of chronic sinusitis are similar to those of acute sinusitis, but they are usually milder and last for longer duration (more than 8 to 12 weeks). These presentations include: nasal congestion and stuffiness, thick nasal discharge, and facial pain at the sites of the sinuses (forehead, around orbits, at cheeks, or at the nose).

CT scan is an important tool in investigating sinusitis. In acute sinusitis, CT scan usually shows air-fluid levels and gases. Chronic sinusitis is characterized by thickening of the mucosa of the affected sinuses with polyps or hypertrophied nasal turbinates. Sometimes, patients have acute sinusitis on top of chronic sinusitis. In these cases, the findings can be a mixture of both types described above. Involvement of one sinus only with hyperdense areas in the opacities inside the sinus should raise the probability of fungal sinusitis.

15. PROGRESSIVE NASAL STUFFINESS AND FACIAL PAIN

A 67-year-old male had a CT scan because he suffered from progressive nasal stuffiness, rhinorrhea, and facial pain. The images below are taken from his CT scan.

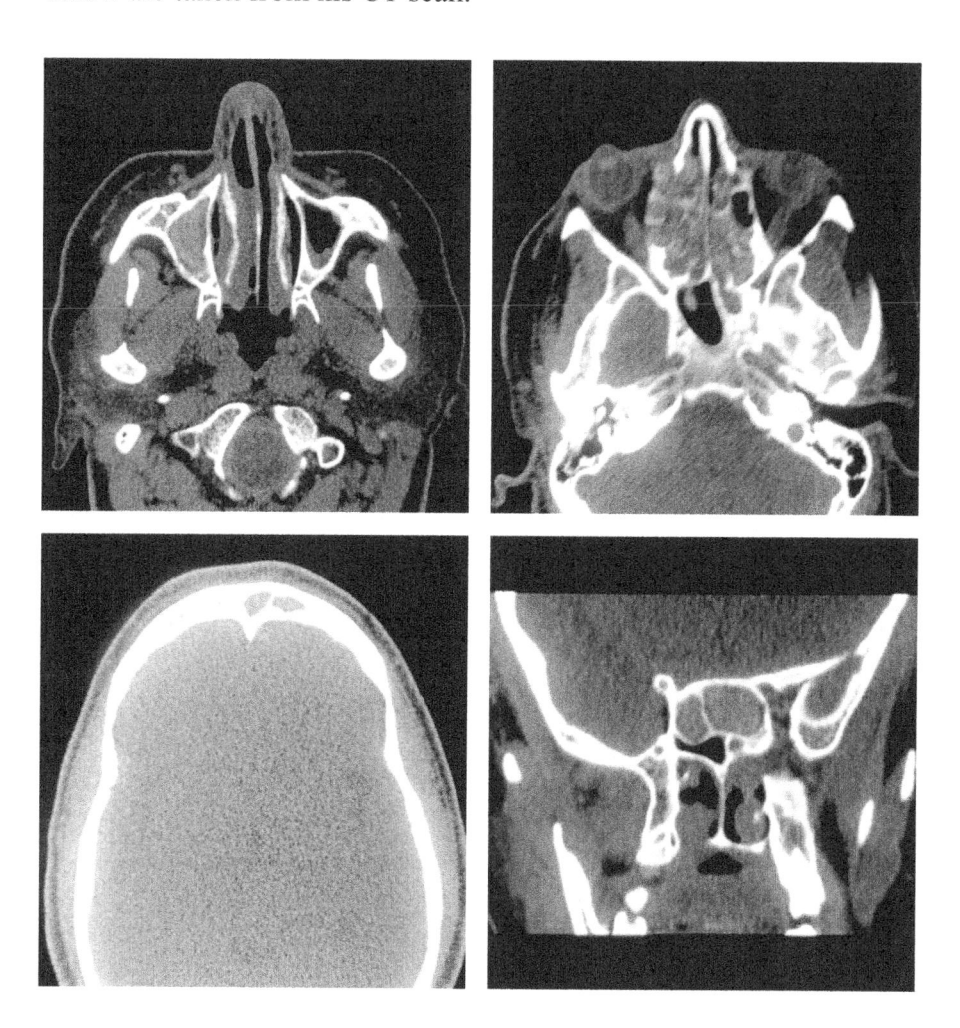

Questions

1. What are the findings seen in this scan?

2. What is the diagnosis?

3. What are the diseases that are commonly associated with this condition?

Answers and Discussion

The CT scan images show multiple polypoidal soft tissue masses in the nasal cavity and paranasal sinuses with subtotal opacification of the nasal cavities and paranasal sinuses with convex lateral wall of the right ethmoid sinus. These findings are consistent with sinonasal polyposis.

There are many conditions that are usually associated with sinonasal polyposis. The most common of these conditions are:

- Asthma
- Allergy
- Cystic fibrosis
- Aspirin insensitivity

Sinonasal polyposis can present with multiple symptom, the most common of these symptoms are:

- Progressive nasal stuffiness
- Rhinorrhea
- Facial pain
- Headache
- Anosmia

Treatment of sinonasal polyposis involves a combination of medical options to manage this condition (such as antibiotics, steroids, and anti-leukotrienes) and surgical procedures. Surgery usually is not the final cure for this condition because of the high recurrence rate.

16. NASAL CONGESTION AND SNORING

An 18-year-old female complains of nasal congestion which is more on the left side and snoring during sleep. The image below is taken from a noncontrast enhanced CT scan that was done to assess her nose and paranasal sinuses.

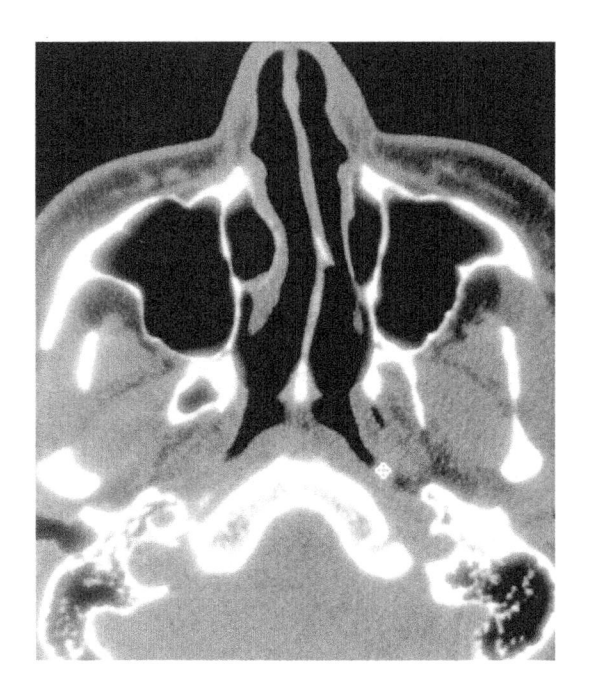

Questions

1. What are the findings seen in this scan?

2. What are the causes of this condition?

3. What are the complications of this condition?

Answers and Discussion

This patient has moderate deviation of the nasal septum to the left side.

Deviation of the nasal septum can be caused by one of many things. The most important of these causes are:

- Congenital deviation
- Trauma to the nose
- Connective tissue disorders (for example, Marfan syndrome and Ehlers–Danlos syndrome).

The most common complications of deviated nasal septum include:

- Sleep disturbance.
- Dry mouth
- Chronic nasal congestion
- Acute and chronic sinusitis

Deviation of the nasal septum is very common. It is estimated that about 80% of humans have nasal septum deviation of some degree. Most of these cases are asymptomatic and the deviation doesn't cause any problems.

When the deviation of the nasal septum causes symptoms, it can present with nasal congestion (usually more on the side of the deviation), recurrent sinusitis, headache, epistaxis, facial pain, and snoring.

The severity of the deviation of the nasal septum can be graded using the grading system proposed by Jin et al. The following table illustrates the grades in that system.

Jin et al. Grading for the severity of nasal septum deviation	
Grade	Description
Mild	Deviation in which the deviated septum crosses less than 50% of the distance between the nasal septum and the lateral wall of the nose.
Moderate	Deviation in which the deviated septum crosses more than 50% of the distance between the nasal septum and the lateral wall of the nose.
Severe	Deviation in which the deviated septum touches the lateral wall of the nose.

The choice of treatment of nasal septum deviation depends on the severity of the symptoms produced by it. In the case of mild symptoms, nasal decongestants, nasal steroid sprays, and antihistamines are enough. In more severe symptoms, surgical correction of the deviation might be needed.

17. ACUTE PAIN IN THE RIGHT EAR WITH HEARING IMPAIRMENT

A 52-year-old female who complains of acute right ear pain had a decreased hearing on the right side on examination and was sent for a CT scan of temporal bones. The images below are taken for her scan.

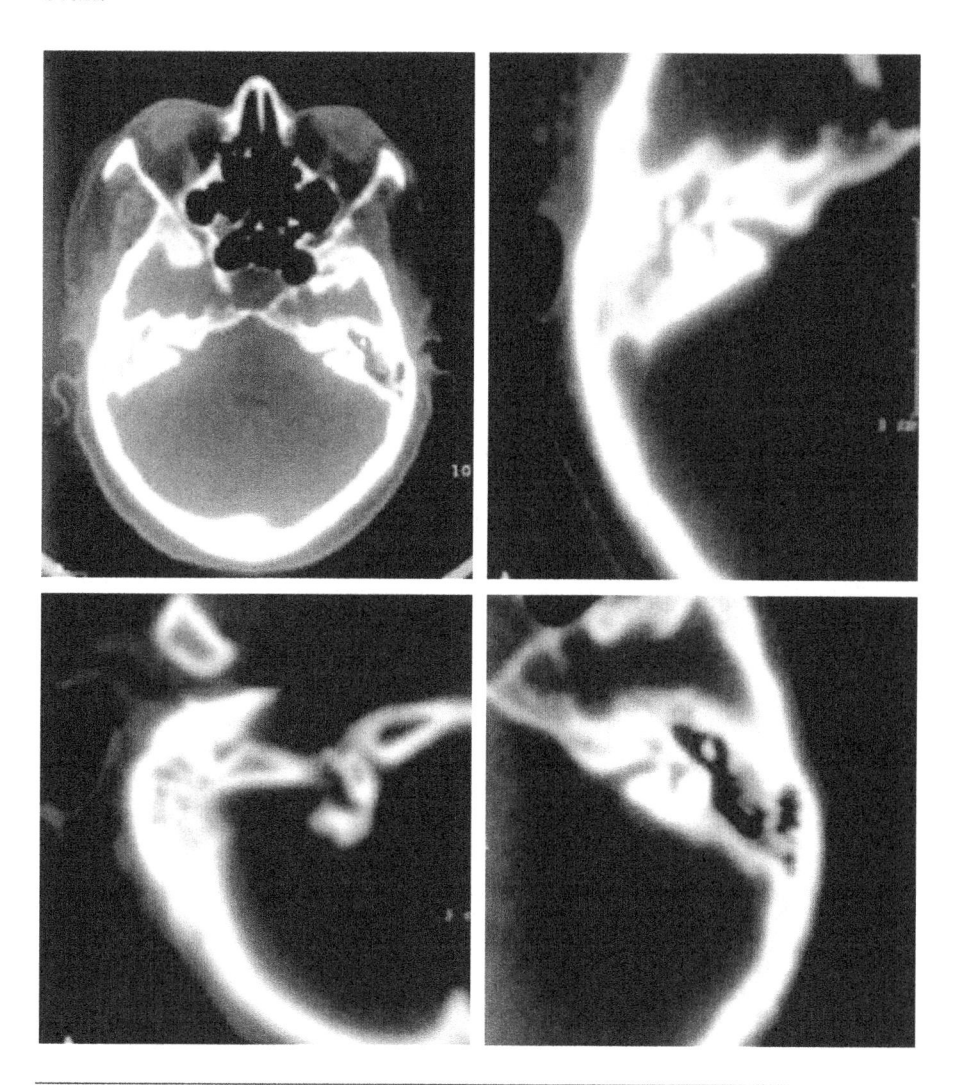

Questions

1. What are the findings seen in this scan?

2. What is the diagnosis?

3. What are the common causes of this condition?

Answers and Discussion

The images show opacification of the right middle ear cavity and mastoid air cells on the right side. These findings are consistent with otitis media and mastoiditis (acute otomastoidits).

Otitis media is a very common infection that affects more than 10% of the population each year. It is the second most common infection in childhood. It can be acute (of a duration that is less than 2 weeks) or chronic (of a duration that is more than 2 weeks). The most common causative organism of otitis media is Streptococcus pneumoniae which causes about half of the causes. Other common causative organisms are Haemophilus influenzae and Moraxella catarrhalis.

The most common presentation of acute otitis media is fever, ear pain and hearing loss or impairment in the affected ear. Usually there is dysfunction of the Eustachian tube that facilitates the middle ear infection. This dysfunction can result from a viral infection of the upper respiratory tract or from allergy. Symptoms in very young children differ from symptoms in adults or older children. Very young children have fever, irritability, poor feeding, and pulling or rubbing of the affected ear. In chronic otitis media, the patient usually presents with recurrent ear pain and hearing impairment.

Acute and chronic otitis media have different appearances on CT scan of temporal bones. In acute otitis media, there is usually opacification of middle ear cavity and mastoid air cells due to fluid collection and sometimes air-fluid level can be seen. Sometimes, bone erosion can occur in acute otitis media and an abscess or fistula can be detected. Chronic otitis media usually results in destruction of middle ear ossicles and bone erosions. In addition to this, calcification and soft tissue debris can be found in middle ear cavity. Destruction and poor aeration of mastoid air cells is a common finding on CT scan in cases of chronic otitis media.

Otitis media have many complications. The most important of these complications are:

- Extracranial complications:
  - Mastoiditis
  - Petrositis
  - Labyrinthitis
  - Labyrinthine fistula
  - Postauricular abscess
  - Temporal abscess
  - Facial palsy
- Intracranial complications:
  - Meningitis
  - Brain abscess
  - Sigmoid sinus thrombosis

18. SLOWY GROWING NECK SWELLING

A 43-year-old female presented with a slowly growing painless anterior neck swelling and normal thyroid functions tests. The images below are taken from contrast-enhanced CT scan of her neck.

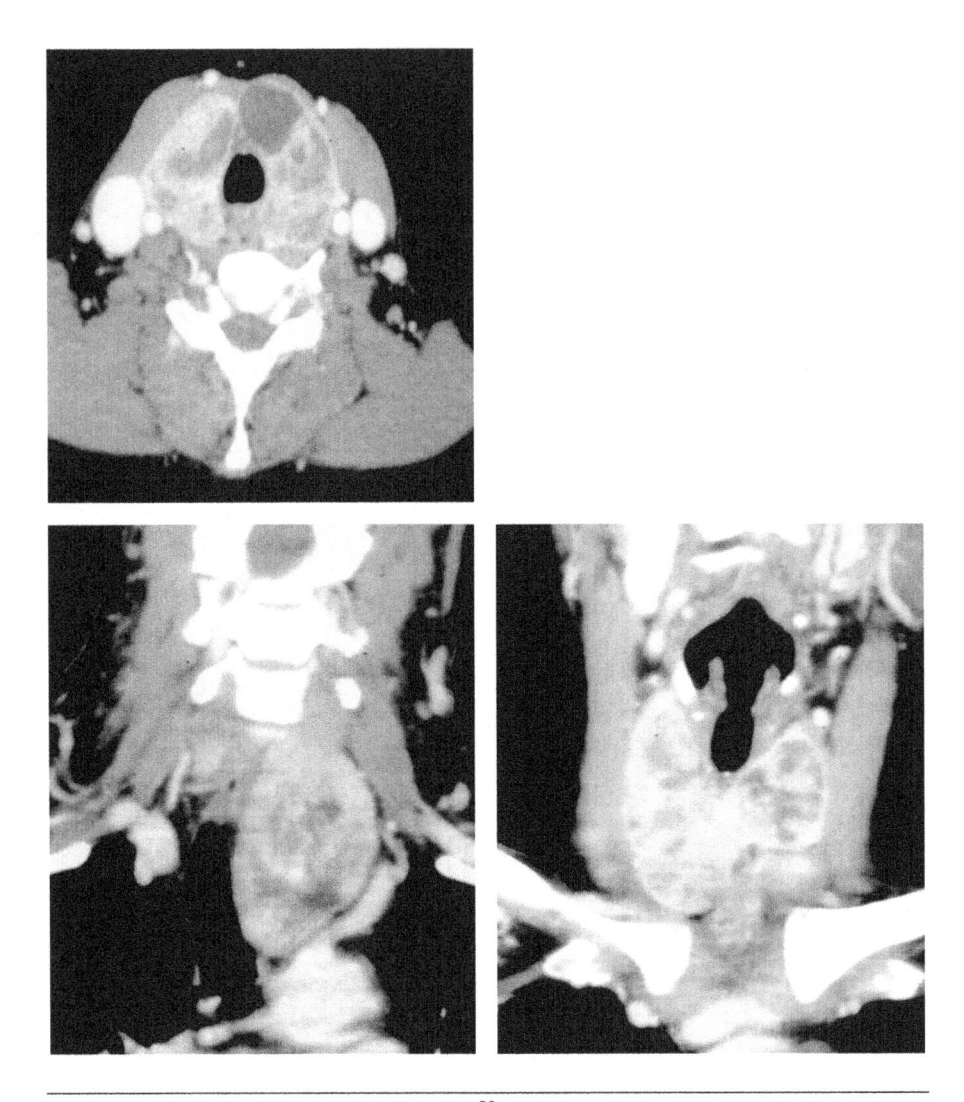

Questions

1. What are the findings seen in this scan?

2. What is the diagnosis?

3. What are the complications of this condition?

Answers and Discussion

The images show heterogeneous enlargement of both lobes of the thyroid gland after contrast administration. These findings are consistent with multinodular goiter. Complications of multinodular goiter include:

- Airways compression causing exertional or positional dyspnea.
- Hoarseness of voice
- Dysphagia
- Superior vena cava compression

Goitre is a term that refers to enlarged thyroid gland. In multinodular goiter, the thyroid gland enlarges and contains multiple nodules. This condition is more common in females between the 4th and 6th decade. Multinodular goiter patients usually have normal thyroid functions, but some of them have hypo- or hyperfunction. Patients with multinodular goiter have increased risk of thyroid cancer (more than 10% of patients with multinodular goiter who undergo surgery have thyroid cancer identified in their glands).

Multinodular goitre has variable presentations:

- Asymptomatic

- Slowly growing neck swelling (for years)
- Symptoms of compression (dyspnea, dysphagia, hoarseness of voice)
- Symptoms of thyrotoxicosis (palpitation, tremors, irritability, etc.)
- Symptoms of hypothyroidism (lethargy, myxedema, constipation, etc.)

World Health Organization (WHO) has a clinical classification for goitre that includes five grades. The following table illustrates these grades:

WHO grading system for Goitre	
Grade	**Description**
Grade 0	Thyroid gland is impalpable or visible
Grade Ia	Thyroid gland is palpable but not visible
Grade Ib	Thyroid gland is palpable in normal position and visible on hyperextension of the neck
Grade II	Thyroid gland is palpable an visible in normal position of the neck
Grade III	Thyroid gland is palpable an is clearly visible from distance

Although CT scan can diagnose multinodular goitre, ultrasonography remains the best modality in diagnosing multinodular goitre, following up the already diagnosed cases, and in guiding fine needle aspiration biopsy of the nodules. The sensitivity of ultrasound in detecting even small nodules is more than 95%. CT scan advantage is that it is very useful for evaluating retrosternal extension of the goitre (something that ultrasound has a limited ability to do).

19. LUNG CAVITATIONS IN A 25-YEAR-OLD MALE

A 25-year-old male came to hospital complaining of chronic cough that started 6 months ago and is associated with night fever and sweats. His history revealed appetite loss and significant weight loss in the last few months. The images below are taken from high resolution CT scan of his chest. .

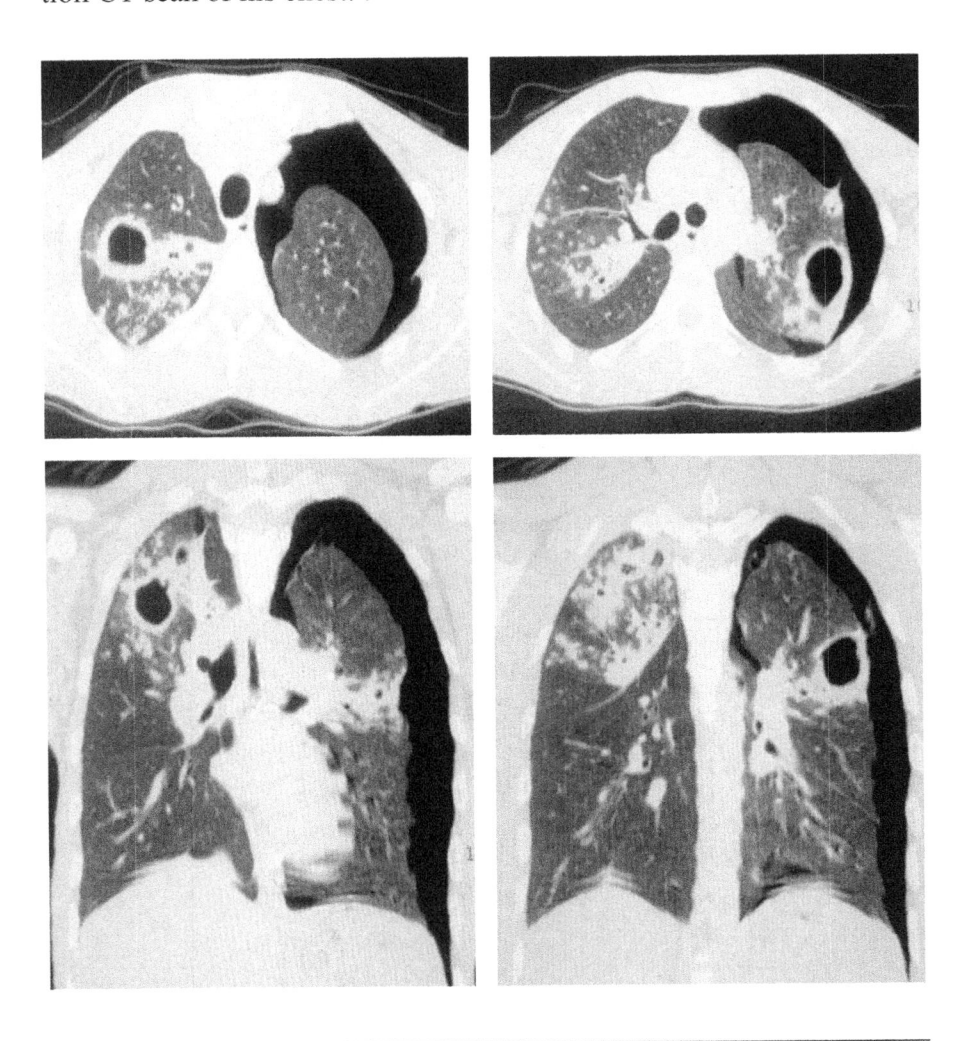

Questions

1. What are the findings seen in this scan?

2. What is the diagnosis?

3. What is the differential diagnosis of cavitary lesions in the lungs?

Answers and Discussion

Two cavitary lesions are seen in the images of the scan. The first is in the upper lobe of left lung and the second is in the upper lobe of the right lung. Both lesions have thick irregular walls. They are surrounded by localized consolidation. A pneumothorax is present on the left side. These findings are consistent with tuberculous pneumonia.

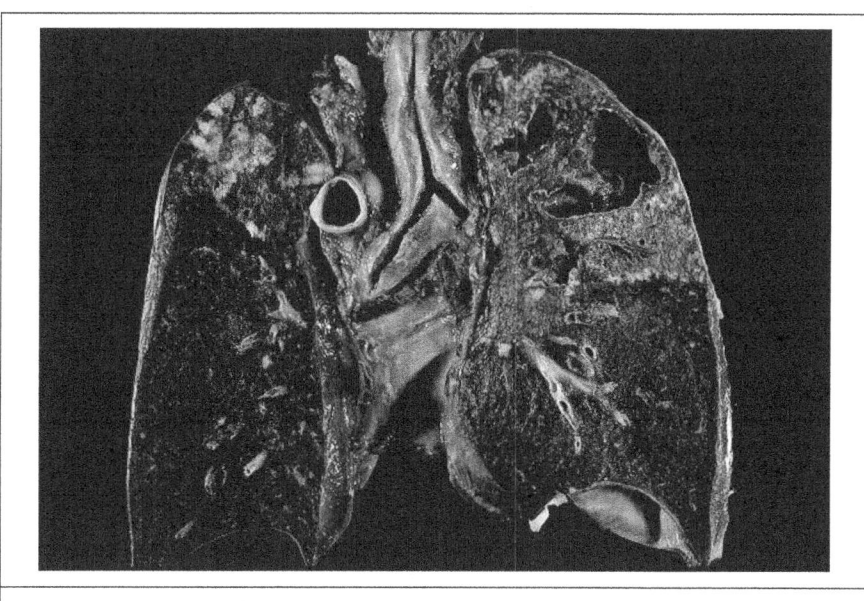

Cavitary tuberculosis

(By Yale Rosen. Licensed under CC BY-SA 2.0.)

The differential diagnosis of cavitary lesions in the lungs includes:

- Malignancies:
  - Bronchogenic carcinoma
  - Metastases
- Infections:
  - Pulmonary Tuberculosis
  - Lung abscess
- Other cases:
  - Rheumatoid Arthritis
  - Bronchogenic cyst

Cavitary lesions are air-filled lesions found in the lung on chest x-ray or CT scan. They can be found within areas of consolidation, nodules, or masses. Differentiation between lung cysts and lung cavitary lesions depends on the wall thickness. Cysts usually have thin walls (4 mm or less) and cavities have thick walls (5 mm or more).

Patients with tuberculous pneumonia present with many symptoms that usually include shortness of breath, chronic cough, hemoptysis, weight loss, appetite loss, night fever, and night sweats. A significant number of patients don't have any symptoms or have only mild symptoms on presentation.

It is important to differentiate cavitary lesions caused by tuberculosis or lung abscess from lesions caused by malignant tumours because cavities are common in lung malignancies and has been detected by CT scan in up to 22% of patients with primary lung cancers in some studies.

Thick walls can suggest malignancy especially if the wall thickness is above 15 mm. other features that can help in identifying malignant cavities are the irregular margins or the presence of the cavity inside a solitary lung nodule. Lesions with wall thickness between 5 and 15 mm can be benign or malignant, while lesions with thin walls are almost always benign.

20. FOUL SMELLING SPUTUM AFTER PNEUMONIA

A 17-year-old female who had pneumonia and was treated by antibiotics less than 4 weeks ago came back to hospital complaining of fever, productive cough with foul smelling sputum, night sweats, and weight loss. The images below are taken from a noncontrast enhanced CT scan of her.

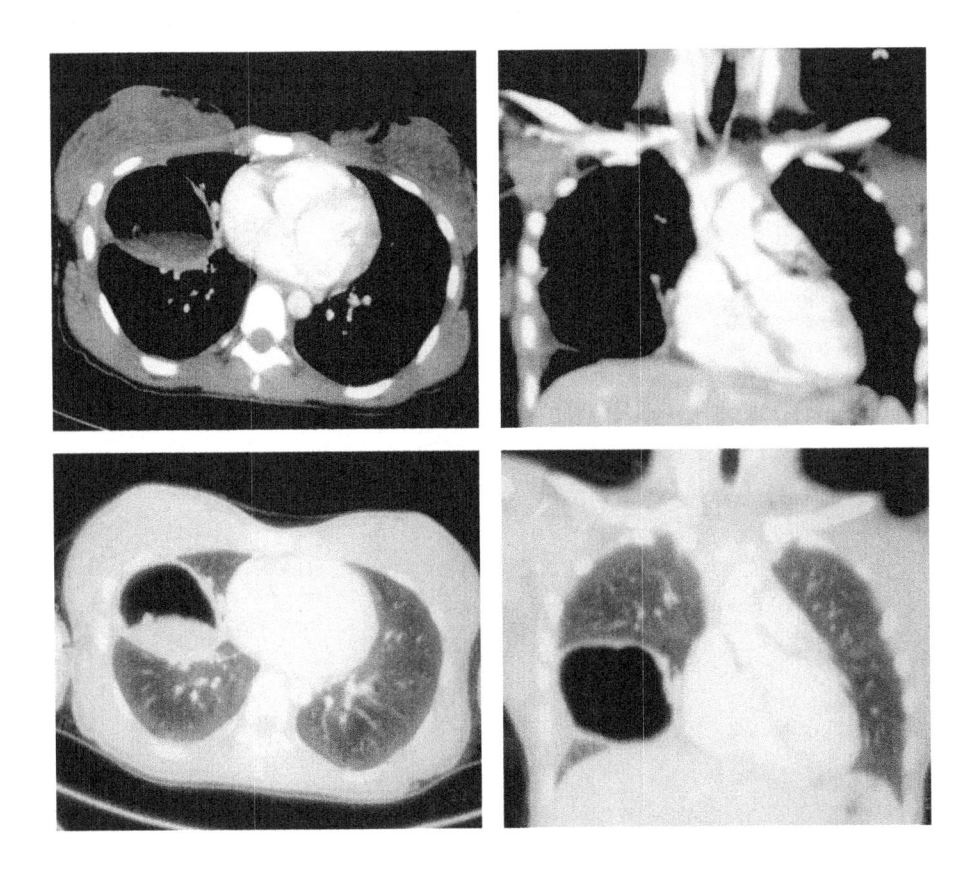

Questions

1. What are the findings seen in this scan?

2. What is the diagnosis?

3. What are the causes of this condition?

Answers and Discussion

The patient images show a cavitary lesion with irregular thin wall in the anterior part of the lower lobe of the right lung. The lesion contains air fluid level. These findings are consistent with a lung abscess.

There are many conditions that can result in the formation of lung abscess. The most common causes are aspiration and endotracheal intubation. The causative organisms are multiple; the most common of them are anaerobic bacteria such as Peptostreptococcus and Bacteroides. Less commonly, lung abscess can be caused by aerobic bacteria such as Staphylococcus, Klebsiella and Haemophilus or by fungi such as Candida and Aspergillus. Amoebic lung abscess can occur as a complication of hepatic amoebiasis.

Lung abscess can occur in any age and even in healthy people, but old people and peoples with malnutrition or who are immunocompromised are more likely to have lung abscess than the general population. In addition to this, people with conditions that can decrease their level of conscious are more likely to aspirate their oral secretions and get aspiration pneumonia and lung abscesses.

Patients with lung abscess can have acute or chronic presentation according the causative organism. Typical presentations include fever, shortness of breath, cough with foul smelling sputum, hemoptysis, and pleuritic chest pain.

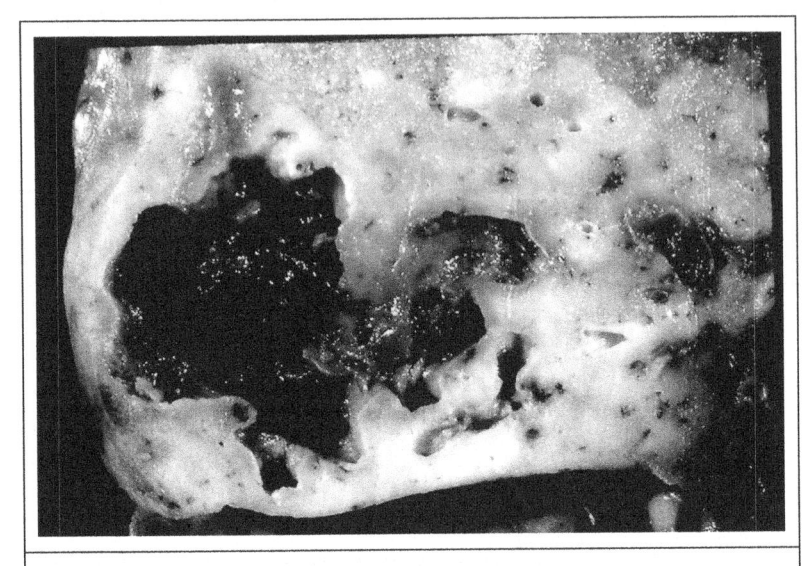

Macroscopic appearance of lung abscess.

(By Yale Rosen. Licensed under CC BY-SA 2.0.)

Differential diagnosis of lung abscess on chest x-ray and CT scan should include other cavitary lung lesions such as TB cavitations and lung cancer. Usually the air-fluid level helps in differentiating lung abscess from other conditions. In addition to this, the clinical presentation of the patient and the wall thickness of the abscess cavity and its regularity and smooth borders can help.

Although lung abscess can respond to antibiotic treatment, it can still be fatal in some cases especially if the patient is immunocompromised (for example AIDS patients) where mortality rate is up to 75% of cases.

21. FEVER, NIGHT SWEATS AND PLEURITIC CHEST PAIN.

The images below are taken from a CT scan that was done for a 45-year-old male patient who complains of high fever and chills, night sweats, and right sided chest pain on inspiration.

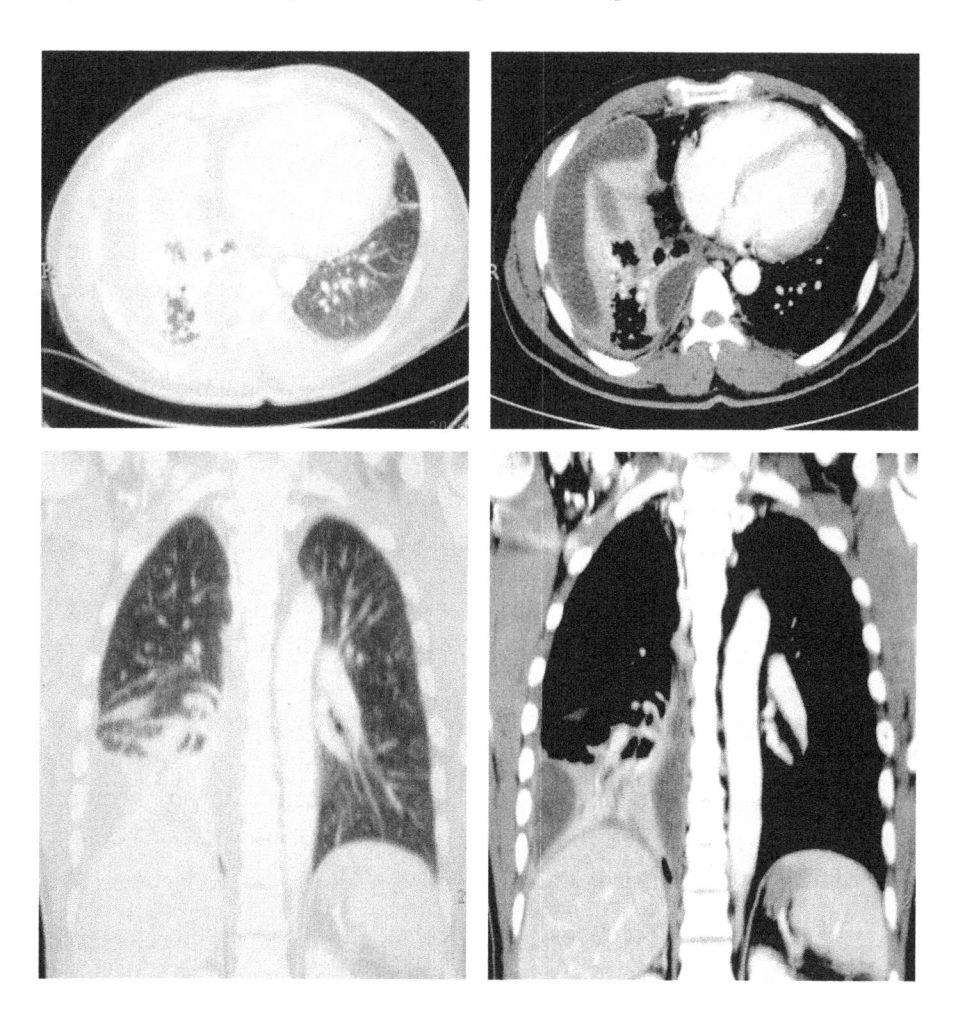

Simple common cases in CT scan

Questions

1. What are the findings seen in this scan?

2. What is the diagnosis?

3. What are the most important differential diagnoses of this condition?

Answers and Discussion

The CT scan images show a fluid density collection in the right pleural space with split pleura sign and small area of consolidation in the lower lobe of the right lung. These findings are consistent with empyema.

The most common differential diagnoses of this condition include:

- Malignant pleural effusion
- Malignant mesothelioma

In empyema, pus collects in a cavity inside the body. Usually the word 'empyema' used to refer to thoracic empyema which is accumulation of pus in the pleural cavity. The difference between empyema and lung abscess is that in empyema, the pus accumulate inside an already present cavity (in cases of thoracic empyema, the cavity is the pleural space), while in lung abscess, the pus accumulates in a newly created space that results from lung tissue necrosis due to inflammation.

Empyema usually results from pneumonia. Other causes of empyema are chest trauma, subdiaphragmatic abscess, and paravertebral abscesses. Rarely empyema occurs after thoracentesis. The most common organisms that cause empyema are Streptococci (milleri and pneumoniae), Staphylococcus aureus, and anaerobic bacteria.

Empyema has three different stages. The first stage is called the acute stage, serous stage, or exudative stage. In this stage, no bacteria can be found in the fluid accumulated in the pleural space. The second stage is called the intermediate stage or fibrinopurulent stage. In this stage, the fluid become infected and bacterial cultures of aspirated fluid are positive. Draining should be done in this stage. In the last stage (which is called the late stage or organizing stage), fibroblasts proliferates and produce a fibrous covering. These stages cannot be differentiated by imaging.

The presentation of empyema is usually non-specific. And it includes symptoms of chest infection such as fever, shortness of breath, cough, loss of appetite, and pleuritic chest pain. In addition to this, the history can show the cause (pneumonia, subdiaphragmatic abscess, chest trauma, etc.). Mortality rate in cases of empyema can reach up to 10%.

22. AN OLD MALE WITH A SOLITARY LUNG NODULE

A 68-year-old male who is a heavy smoker had a lung nodule on a chest x-ray that he had during a routine checkup. The images below are taken from High resolution CT scan of his chest.

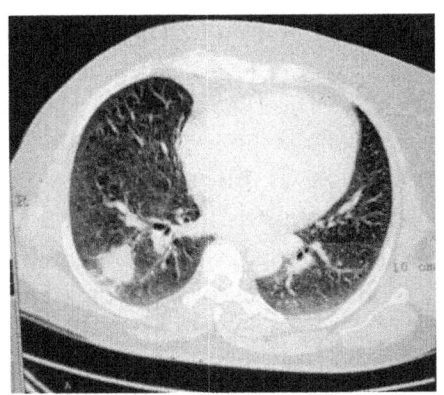

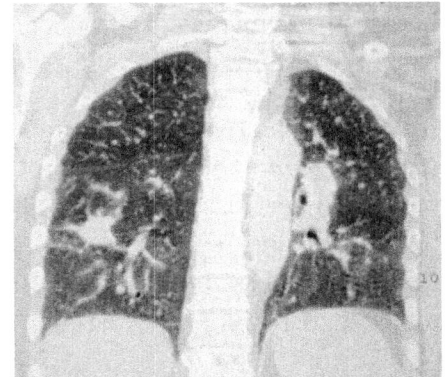

Questions

1. What are the findings seen in this scan?

2. What is the diagnosis?

3. What is the differential diagnosis of a solitary lung nodule?

Answers and Discussion

The images show a well-defined nodule with speculated edges in the middle lobe of right lung with no evidence of calcification. This finding is consistent with bronchogenic carcinoma.

The differential diagnosis of a solitary pulmonary nodule includes a long list of causes. These are usually classified as malignant and benign conditions (like hamatomas, infection, inflammations, etc.). The table below lists the most important of these causes:

Differential diagnosis of a solitary pulmonary nodule			
Neoplastic	**Infectious**	**Inflammatory**	**Others**
• Carcinoma • Metastasis • Lymphoma • hamartoma	• Lung abscess • Hydatid cyst	• Rheumatoid arthritis • Sarcoidosis	• Bronchogenic cyst • Lung infarction

The most common type of malignancies is lung cancer, and about 80-90% of lung cancer cases are related to smoking. Lung cancers are classified into:

- Non-small-cell lung cancer
    - Squamous cell carcinoma
    - Adenocarcinoma
    - Large-cell carcinoma
- Small-cell lung cancer

The presentations of lung carcinoma are variable and can be generally classified into three groups of presentations:

- Presentations related to the tumour itself:
    - Shortness of breath
    - Hemoptysis
    - Wheeze or stridor
    - Pleuritic chest pain
- Presentations related to metastasis:
    - Headache, vomiting
    - Bone pain and pathological fractures

- Upper abdominal pain and jaundice
- Presentations related to the paraneoplastic syndrome:
  - Cushing syndrome
  - Hypercalcemia
  - Hyponatremia
  - Clubbing and hypertrophic pulmonary osteoarthropathy

Lung carcinoma can have variable appearances on chest x-ray and chest CT scans. It can present as a nodule, a cavitary lesion, or an alveolar effusion. It can also be associated with some of its complications such as pneumonia, bronchiectasis, or collapse of a lung or a lung segment.

When a solitary nodule is found on imaging, it is important to detect and describe benign and malignancy suggesting features. The size of the nodule is an important feature. In general, small nodules (less than 5 mm in size) are rarely malignant, while larger nodules tend to be malignant (about half of the nodules that are 2 cm and larger are malignant). Most malignant nodules have speculated irregular margins. When a cavity appears with the nodule, the site of the cavity and the thickness of the wall of the cavity can help in differentiating malignant from benign nodules. In malignant nodules, the cavities are usually central and the wall of the cavity is thick and irregular.

23. CHRONIC COUGH AND SHORTNESS OF BREATH

A 39-year-old female with chronic cough and shortness of breath was found to have rhonchi and crepitiation in the middle and lower zones of both lungs on auscultation. A high resolution CT scan of chest was done. The images below are taken from her scan.

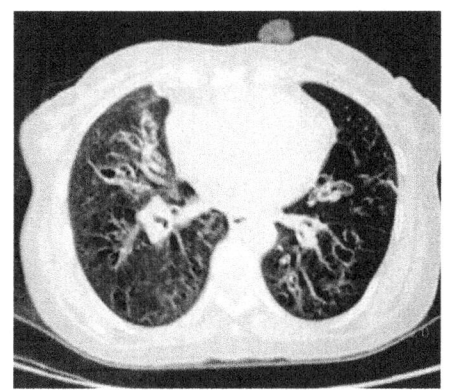

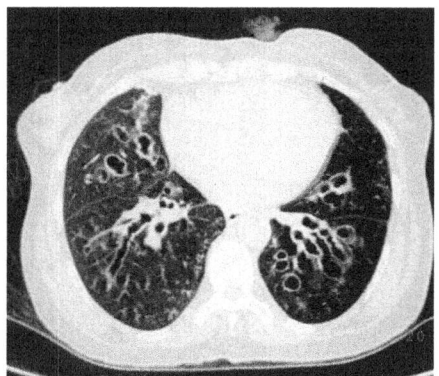

Questions

1. What are the findings seen in this scan?

2. What is the diagnosis?

3. What are the causes of this condition?

Answers and Discussion

The images show diffuse lesions in both lungs in the form of dilatation in the bronchial tree with variable diameters of the dilated bronchi and beaded appearance of their outlines. This finding is consistent with Bronchiectasis of moderate severity (varicose type).

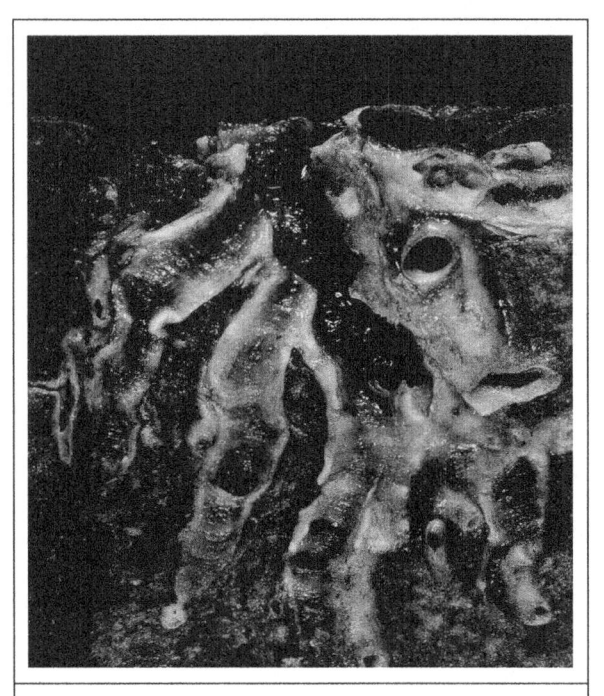

Bronchiectasis

(By Dr Yale Rosen. Licensed under CC BY-SA 2.0.)

Bronchiectasis is an obstructive lung disease that is characterized by irreversible dilation of the bronchial tree. It can result from congenital or acquired causes:

- Acquired causes:
  - pneumonia (bacterial, tuberculous, measles)

- obstruction of bronchial tree (by a foreign body or a tumor)
- Congenital causes:
  - Cystic fibrosis
  - Kartagener syndrome
  - Alpha-1-antitrypsin deficiency

Patients with bronchiectasis can present in various ways. Some of them present with shortness of breath and productive cough while others present with hemoptysis only. On auscultation of the chest, there are usually crepitations and/or rhonchi.

Based on the findings on pathological examination of lungs and CT scan findings, Bronchiectasis can be graded or classified into one of the three grades. The following table explains this grading.

Grading or classification of bronchiectasis		
Grade	Names	Description
Mild	Cylindrical (tubular)	In this type, the diameter of the bronchi is uniform.
Moderate	Varicose	This type has dilated bronchi with beaded walls.
Severe	Cystic (saccular)	This is the most severe form of bronchiectasis. In this type, there is cyst-like dilatation of bronchi with air-fluid level seen inside them. The diameter of these cysts can reach up to 3 centimeter

24. AN INCIDENTAL SUBCUTANEOUS MASS IN THE BACK

The images below are taken from CT scan of chest of a 52-year-old male who was suspected to have lung fibrosis on a routine pre-operative chest x-ray.

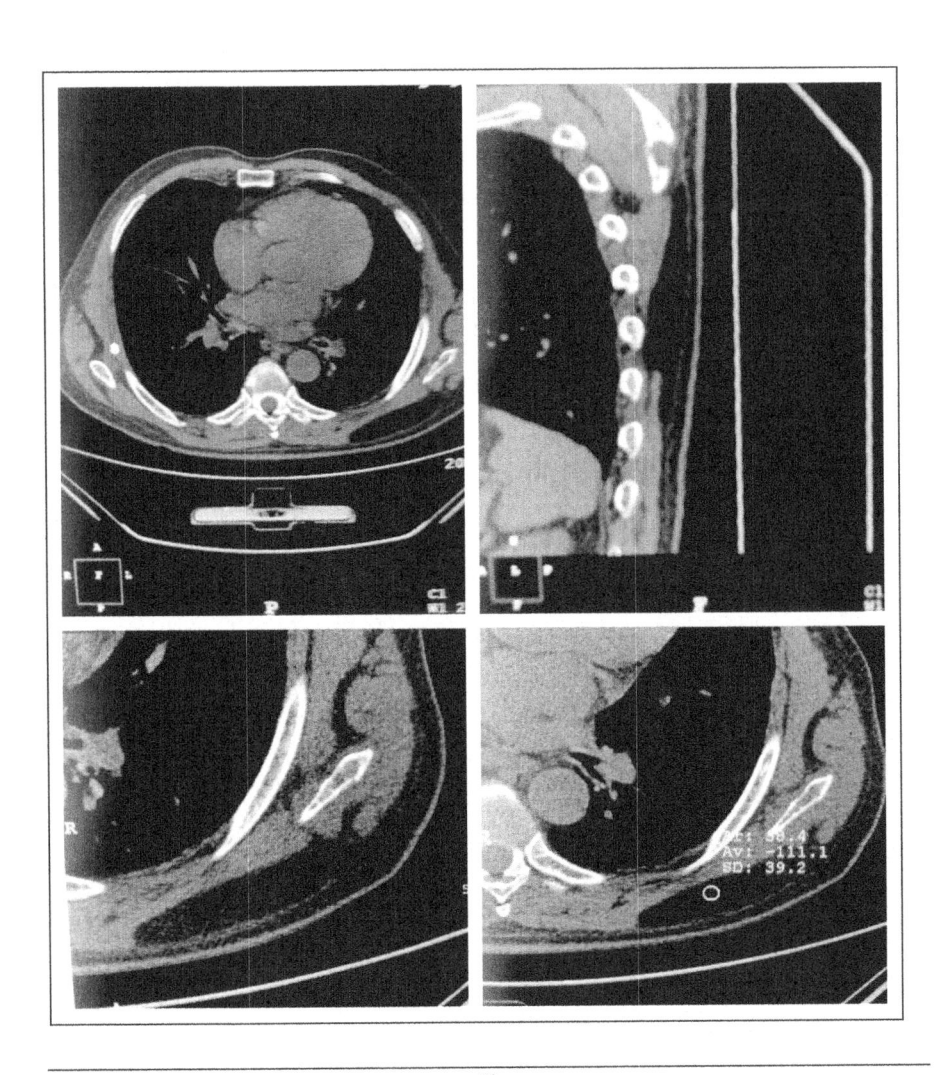

Questions

1. What are the findings seen in this scan?

2. What is the diagnosis?

3. What are the most important differential diagnoses for this condition?

Answers and Discussion

The images show a well-defined homogenous fat-density mass in the subcutaneous tissue of the back medial to the left scapula. These findings are consistent with a subcutaneous lipoma.

The most important differential diagnoses of chest wall lipoma are:

- Liposarcoma
- Pleural lipoma
- Spindle cell lipoma
- Lipoblastoma

Lipomas are the most common benign connective tissues tumors. They can be found in any age group, but they are most commonly found in elderly and obese patients. Lipomas are more common in males than in females.

Clinically they present as palpable mobile soft tissue masses. Their size is variable and they can reach up to 10 centimeters or more. Usually they are single, but in rare cases they can be multiple. When they are large, they can compress the surrounding structures.

Lipomas can be found anywhere in the body except in the brain, eye lids, and penis. They can be classified according to their site into: subcutaneous, intramuscular, intraglandular, subperiosteal, extradural, subsynovial, submucous, and subserous lipomas.

On CT scan, they are seen as well-defined homogenous fat density soft tissue lesions. Their density ranges from -65 to -120 Hounsfield units. If contrast is used, they show no enhancement.

When they are larger than 10 centimeters or they are found in males older than seventy years old, or they contain thick septations or when calcification is seen inside them, then the diagnosis of Liposarcoma should be considered. When they take any contrast, then suspicion should be raised and other diagnoses should be sought.

25. A CYSTIC LIVER LESION ON ULTRASOUND

A 39-year old male is complaining from an epigastric pain for the last 7 months but with no jaundice or fever. On clinical examination, he had a palpable enlarged liver. He underwent an ultrasonography of the abdomen. Ultrasound has shown a large cyst in the liver. The images below are taken from his contrast-enhanced CT scan.

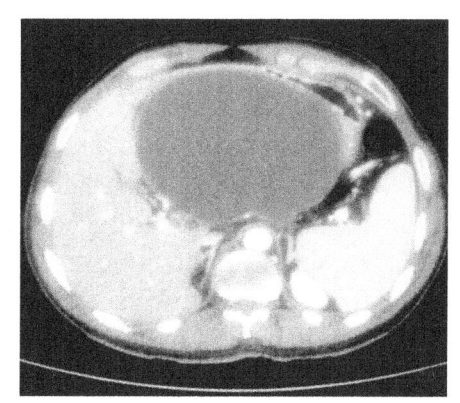

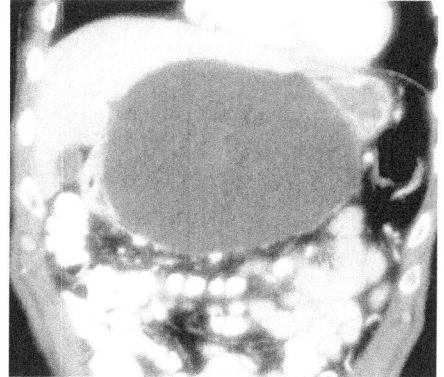

Questions

1. What are the findings seen in this scan?

2. What is the differential diagnosis of a cystic lesion in the liver?

3. What are the causes of this condition?

Answers and Discussion

The images show a large well-defined cystic lesion in the left lobe of liver. The lesion has no septations, mural nodules, or solid component. The wall of the lesion is thin, smooth and regular. There is no enhancement on contrast administration.

Differential diagnoses of solitary cystic lesion in the liver include:

- Simple cysts
- Hydatid cysts
- Liver abscess
- Biloma
- Biliary Cystadenomas or cystadenocarcinoma

Simple liver cysts have variable sizes, ranging from few millimeters up to 10 centimeters. They are usually asymptomatic and are incidentally discovered. They are usually multiple but sometimes they can be solitary. Simple liver cysts can be found in up to 5% of general population and they are benign and don't require any treatment. On noncontrast enhanced CT scan, they appear as well-defined round or oval lesions and after contrast administration they don't take any contrast and show no enhancement. They don't have thick walls, septations, mural nodules or solid component. When their number is more than 10 cysts, the possibility of polycystic liver disease should be considered.

Hydatid cysts are caused by Echinococcus granulosus, Echinococcus multilocularis, and Echinococcus alveolaris. On CT scan, they appear as multiloculated cyst with thick wall and septations. Calcification can be seen inside the daughter cysts sometimes. The size of hydatid cysts is variable and can reach up to 50 centimeters. On contrast administration, there is enhancement of the cyst walls and septations.

Liver abscess can be pyogenic (caused by bacteria) or amoebic (caused by Entamoeba histolytica). Patients with pyogenic abscesses usually present with right upper quadrant pain and fever. On CT scan, pyogenic abscesses appear as multiloculated cystic lesions with enhancement of their walls and septations on contrast administration. Cluster of grapes sign is diagnostic for these abscesses. This sign is formed by the union of small abscess cavities to form one large cavity full of pus. The presence of air is another diagnostic sign, but is not present in all cases. Patients with amebic liver abscesses usually present with right upper quadrant pain with mucous-containing diarrhea. On CT scan, the abscess is usually solitary and shows peripheral (rim) enhancement on contrast administration.

Bilomas are localized collections of bile after a trauma or a surgery. They can be intra- or extrahepatic. On CT scan, they appear as an oval or crescent-shaped fluid collection. After contrast administration, they show no enhancement.

Biliary Cystadenomas are rare benign tumours usually seen in middle-aged females. They can be intra- or extrahepatic. When they are intrahepatic, they are usually seen in the right lobe of liver. They appear as multiloculated cysts with contrast enhancement of the walls and septations. When malignant transformation occurs in biliary cystadenoma, biliary cystadenocarcinoma occurs. The treatment of choice for both of these tumours is complete resection.

26. AN EPIGASTRIC MASS AND WEIGHT LOSS

A 63-year-old male with progressive weight loss for the last 6 months and distension in his upper abdomen had an ultrasound examination that showed a large mass in the liver. His live functions were abnormal and a contrast enhanced CT scan of his abdomen was requested. The images below are taken from his CT scan.

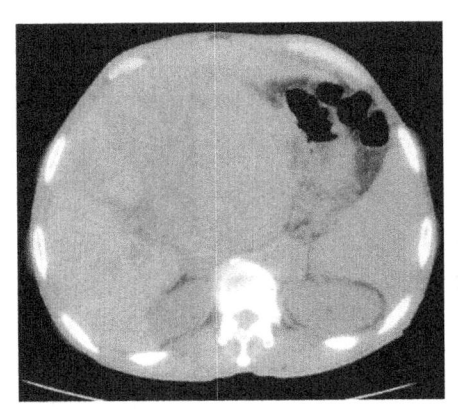

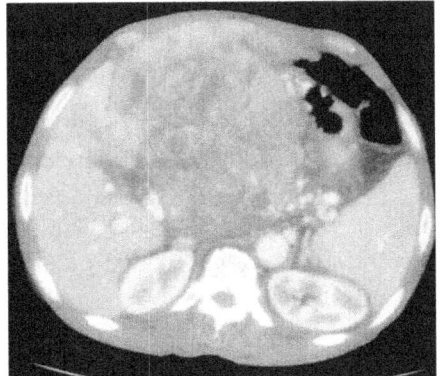

Questions

1. What are the findings seen in this scan?
2. What is the differential diagnosis of a liver mass?

Answers and Discussion

The images show an ill-defined large isodense mass in the left lobe of liver. The mass shows a heterogeneous enhancement on contrast administration.

The differential diagnosis of a liver mass includes:

- Hemangioma
- Metastases
- Hepatocellular carcinoma
- Adenoma
- Focal nodular hyperplasia

Hemanigomas are the most common benign liver tumours. They grow slowly. Their size is variable and they can grow to reach up to 20 centimeters in some cases. On nonenhaced CT scan, they appear as well defined isodense lesions in comparison to the blood vessels of the liver. When they are large, they appear heterogeneous and they might contain a central scar. On contrast administration, they show peripheral nodular enhancement in the arterial phase. The enhancement progresses in the venous phase until the lesion becomes isodense to the blood vessels in the venous and delayed phases. If there is a central scar in the Hemangioma, it doesn't enhance even in the delayed phase.

Metastasis to the liver is very common, and hepatic metastases are the most common malignant tumors in the liver. They can come from any other malignant tumour in the body. When noncontrast enhanced CT scan is done, hepatic metastases appear as multiple hypo-, hyper- or isodense focal lesions in both lobes of liver. Their appearance after contrast administration depends on their vascularity. Hypovascular metastases have peripheral enhancement on the arterial phase while hypervascular metastases have homogenous enhancement in the arterial phase (or heterogeneous enhancement it the tumour contains areas of necrosis). In the venous phase, the tumors become iso- or hypodense.

Hepatocellular carcinomas are the most common primary malignant liver tumour. They represent up to 90% of the primary liver tumours found in adults. Usually they arise in the cases of liver cirrhosis due to any cause. On noncontrast enhanced CT scan, they appear as a single or multiple iso- or hypodense focal lesions. After contrast administration, they show wedge-shaped heterogeneous enhancement in the arterial phase. Their density decreases in the portal venous phase and they become hypodense in comparison to the surrounding liver tissues in the delayed phase.

Hepatic adenomas are rare benign tumours that occur usually in women who use oral contraceptive pills or men who use anabolic steroids. On noncontrast enhanced CT scan, they appear as well-defined iso- or hypodense focal lesions that might contain hyperdense areas of hemorrhage or calcifications or hypodense areas of fat. Their size can reach up to 30 centimeters. After contrast administration, they show heterogeneous enhancement in the arterial phase. The enhancement decreases in the venous phase and disappears in delayed phase.

Focal nodular hyperplasias are rare benign tumors of liver. They are usually small (less than 5 centimeters). They are more common in females in their 3rd to 6th decade of age. Before contrast administration, they appear as well-defined iso- or hypodense focal lesions. After contrast administration, they show strong homogenous enhancement in the arterial phase. In the portal phase, they become iso- or hypodense and in the delayed phase. They finally become isodense in the delayed phase and if they contain a central scar the scar appears hyperdense.

27. ACUTE EPIGASTRIC PAIN AND VOMITING

A 42-year-old alcoholic male was brought to hospital because he is having severe epigastric pain and vomiting. The images below are taken from his contrast-enhanced CT scan of abdomen and pelvis.

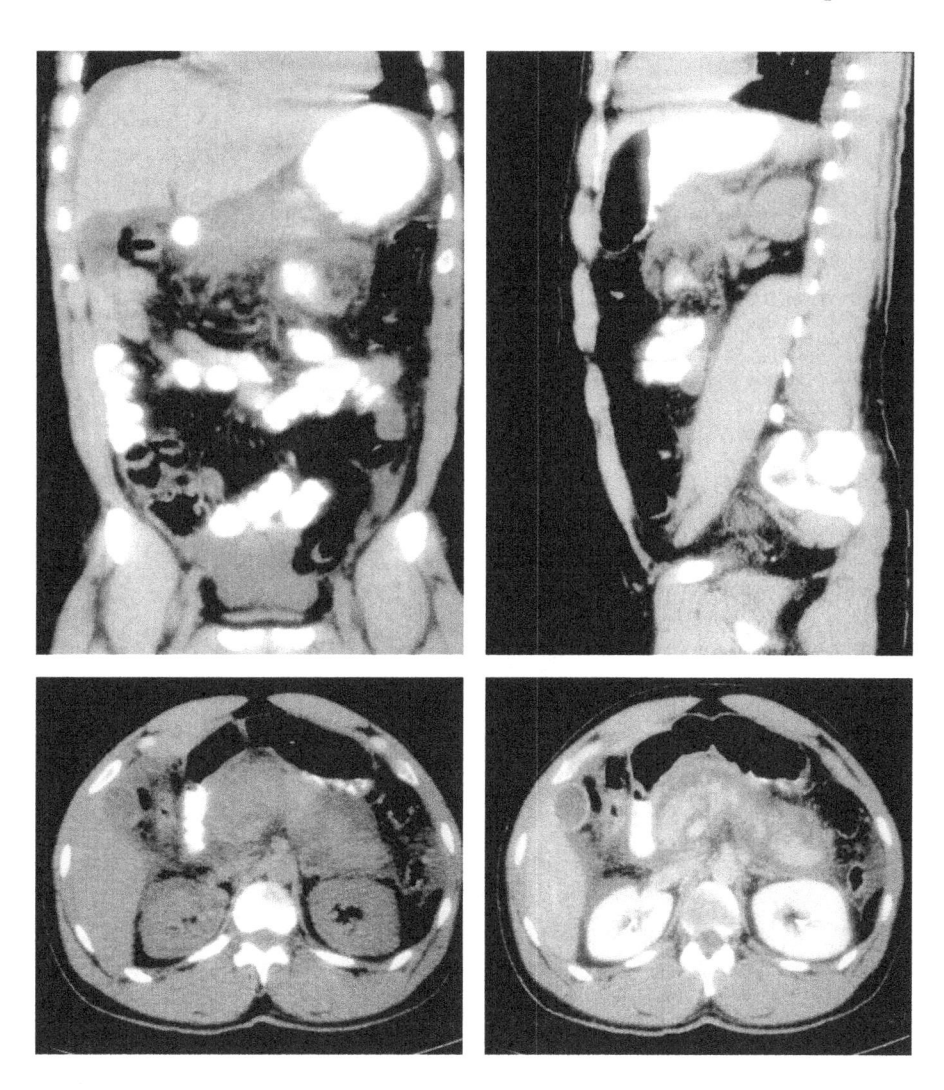

Questions

1. What are the findings seen in this scan?

2. What is the diagnosis?

3. What are the complications of this condition?

Answers and Discussion

The images show diffuse swelling of the pancreas with ill-defined margins and dirty peripancreatic fat. A small amount of peripancreatic fluid is seen. These findings are consistent with acute pancreatitis.

Acute pancreatitis has many complications. The most important of these complications are:

- Local complications:
    o Pseudocyst formation.
    o Abscess formation.
    o Necrosis of the pancreas.
    o Hemorrhage due to vessel erosion.
    o Chronic pancreatitis or even the recurrence of the acute inflammation.
- Systemic complications:
    o Acute Respiratory Distress Syndrome (ARDS).
    o Disseminated Intravascular Coagulation (DIC)
    o Diabetes

There are many causes of acute pancreatitis, but the most common two are gallstones (in 60% of cases) and alcohol (in 30% of cases). Other causes include metabolic abnormalities (hypercalcemia or hyperlipidemia) and different types of injuries (trauma, ERCP), and

Mumps. Some drugs (for example, steroids and OCP) and toxins (snake venoms) are also known to cause acute pancreatitis. In addition to this, some cases of acute pancreatitis are idiopathic.

The most common presentation of acute pancreatitis is severe upper abdominal pain (usually epigastric pain) that radiates to the back and is associated with nausea and vomiting. One examination, multiple findings are usually present. Those findings include abdominal tenderness and guarding, fever, and absent bowel sounds. Less common findings that depend on the type of pancreatitis or its complications include jaundice, dyspnea and, some of the rare signs of (Cullen sign and Grey-Turner sign).

CT scanning is not usually done in cases of acute pancreatitis unless the case is severe or the diagnosis is uncertain. Acute pancreatitis can be graded according to the system created by Balthazar et al. This system is composed of 5 grades (from A to E) and is shown in the table below.

Balthazar et al. system for grading acute pancreatitis based on the findings on CT scan	
Grade	**Description**
Grade A	Normal pancreas
Grade B	Focal or diffuse gland enlargement
Grade C	Intrinsic gland abnormality recognized by haziness on the scan
Grade D	Single ill-defined collection or phlegmon
Grade E	Two or more ill-defined collections or the presence of gas in or nearby the pancreas

28. PAINLESS OBSTRUCTIVE JAUNDICE

A 55-year-old male presented with yellowish discoloration of skins and mucus membranes. His clinical examination showed enlarged liver and jaundice, his investigations has shown obstructive pattern of jaundice. The images below are from contrast-enhanced CT scan of abdomen that the patient had.

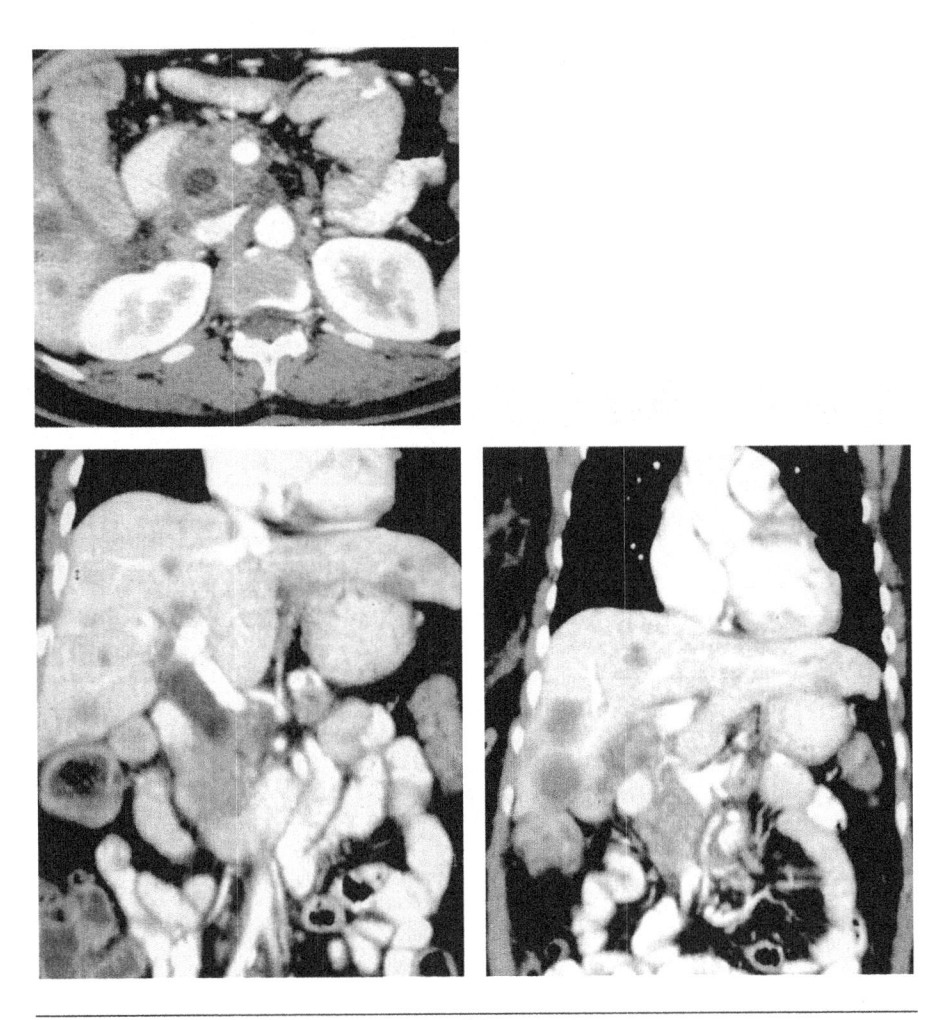

Questions

1. What are the findings seen in this scan?

2. What is the diagnosis?

3. What are the causes of this condition?

Answers and Discussion

The images show an ill-defined mass at the head of pancreas with dilatation of the common bile duct and multiple hypodense lesions in the liver. The liver lesions have weak enhancement on contrast administration. These findings are consistent with cancer of the head of pancreases with live metastasis.

The most common sites for pancreatic tumors are the head and neck of pancreas. About 75% of all pancreatic tumors occur in these regions. Pancreatic tumours can present in many ways, but most of them are non-specific. The most specific presentation for pancreatic tumors is painless obstructive jaundice. Other presentations include pruritus, weight loss, and diabetes mellitus.

The most common types of pancreatic tumours that arise at the head of pancreas include:

- Ductal adenocarcinoma
- Intraductal papillary mucinous neoplasms (IPMNs)
- Serous cystadenoma of the pancreas
- Pancreatoblastomas

Of the four tumours mentioned above, the first one is solid and is the most common and represents about 90% of all pancreatic tumours. The next two are cystic tumours and are rare. The last one is a pediatric tumor.

CT scan can be very useful in staging pancreatic tumor. The most commonly used staging system is the TNM system which can be found in the two tables below.

	TNM classes of a pancreatic tumor
	**T categories (The primary tumor)**
	TX	Primary tumor cannot be assessed
	T0	No evidence of primary tumor
	Tis	Carcinoma in situ
	T1	Tumor limited to the pancreas, ≤ 2 cm in greatest dimension
	T2	Tumor limited to the pancreas, > 2 cm in greatest dimension
	T3	Tumor extends beyond the pancreas but without involvement of the celiac axis or the superior mesenteric artery
	T4	Tumor involves the celiac axis or the superior mesenteric artery (unresectable primary tumor)
	**N categories (Spread to lymph nodes)**
	NX	Regional lymph nodes cannot be assessed
	N0	No regional lymph node metastasis
	N1	Regional lymph node metastasis
	**M categories (Metastasis)**
	M0	No distant metastasis
	M1	Distant metastasis

After determining the T, N and M category of the tumor, the tumor can be put in one of the following anatomical stages:

\multicolumn{5}{c}{Stage grouping of a pancreatic tumor}
Stage	**Substage (if present)**	**T**	**N**	**M**
Stage 0		Tis	N0	M0
Stage I	Stage IA	T1	N0	M0
	Stage IB	T2	N0	M0
Stage II	Stage IIA	T3	N0	M0
	Stage IIB	T1 T2 T3	N1 N1 N1	M0 M0 M0
Stage III		T4	Any N	M0
Stage IV		Any T	Any N	M1

29. AN OLD MAN WITH PAINLESS HEMATURIA

A 72-year-old male presented with painless hematuria of two weeks duration and progressive weight loss for the last 7 months. Ultrasonography has shown an ill-defined mass in the right kidney. The images below are taken from a CT study of his abdomen and pelvis before and after the administration of IV contrast material.

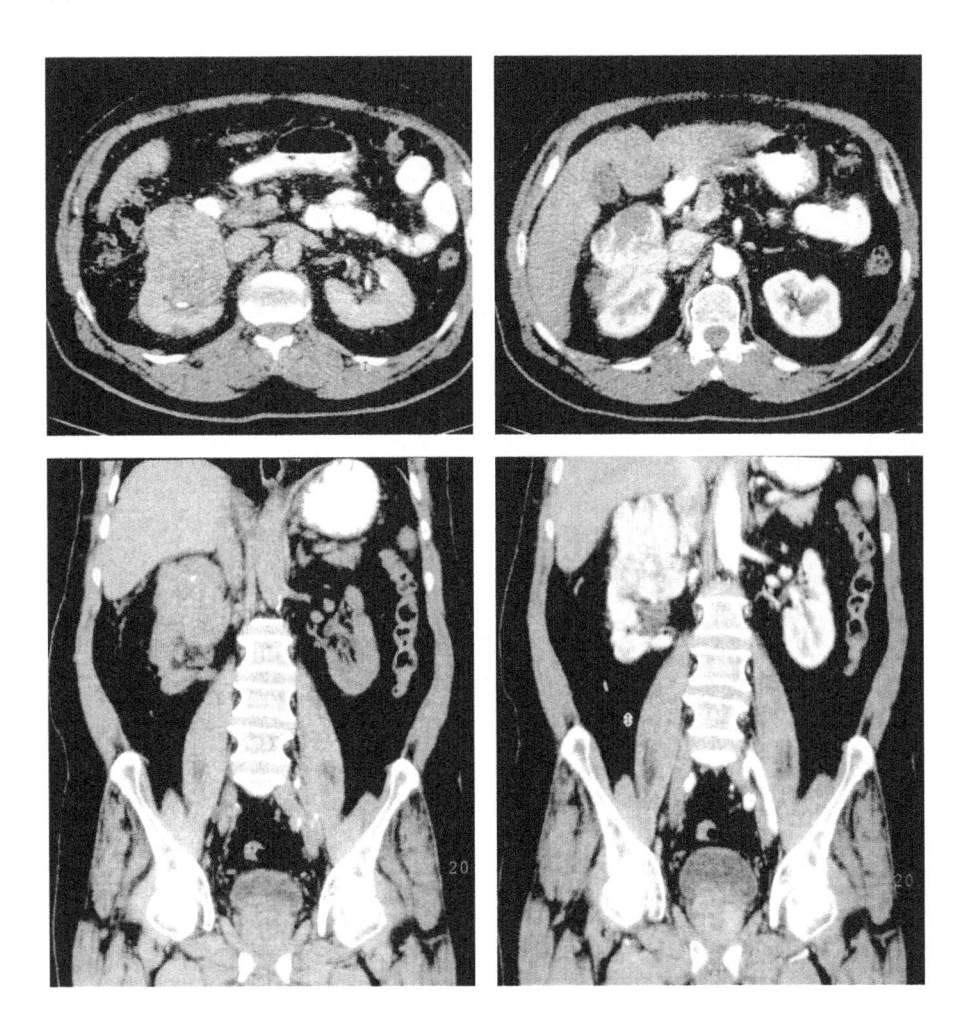

Questions

1. Describe the abnormal finding in the patient's CT scan.

2. What is the most likely diagnosis?

3. What is the differential diagnosis of this finding?

Answers and Discussion

The images show an ill-defined isodense mass in the upper pole of the right kidney. The mass contains small areas of calcification. After administration of contrast, the lesions shows strong heterogeneous enhancement. These findings are consistent with renal cell carcinoma.

Differential diagnoses of a renal mass found in an adult include:

- Benign neoplasms:
    o Renal adenoma
    o Renal oncocytoma
- Malignant neoplasms:
    o Renal cell carcinoma
    o Medullary carcinoma
- Pseudotumours:
    o Prominent column of Bertin
    o Persistent foetal lobulation
    o Renal abscess

Renal cell carcinoma is the most common tumor of the kidney, and it represents about 90-95% of all renal tumors. That is why any renal mass is usually considered renal cell carcinoma until proven otherwise in the day to day practice.

The most common age group having this tumor is people in their 6th to 8th decade. Textbooks describe a classical triad that patients with renal cell carcinoma used to present with. This triad includes hematuria, flank pain, and a palpable mass in the flank. Currently, more than 50% of patients diagnosed with renal cell carcinoma are people in whom the tumor was discovered incidentally. Other symptoms patients might have are fever and weight loss. They might also have hypertension and varicocele.

CT scan is the one of the best imaging modalities for diagnosing renal cell carcinomas and for staging them. The following table shows the different stages of renal cell carcinoma according to the TNM staging system.

Stages of renal cell carcinoma				
Stage	Tumor size	Lymph node involvement	Distant metastasis	Notes
Stage 1	≤ 7 cm	No	No	
Stage 2	≥ 7cm, but still limited to kidney	No	No	
Stage 3	Any size		No	Tumours that reached fatty tissue that surrounds kidney or the large vessels with no

				lymph nodes involvement or metastasis to organs are considered to be stage 3 tumours also.
Stage 4	Any size	Yes (one or more lymph node near the kidney or any distant lymph node)	Yes	Tumours that have spread through fatty tissue around the kidney are considered as stage 4 tumours.

30. AN ADULT FEMALE WITH RIGHT ILLIAC FOSSA PAIN

A 25-year-old female had a central abdominal pain that lasted for few hours 2 days ago and then was followed by sharp stabbing right illiac fossa pain. The pain was associted with anorexia and mild fever. When she came to hospital three days after the onset of the pain, she had leukocytosis and severe tenderness and guarding in the right illiac fossa. Her temperature become 39°C. The images below are taken from her CT scan of the abdomen and pelvis.

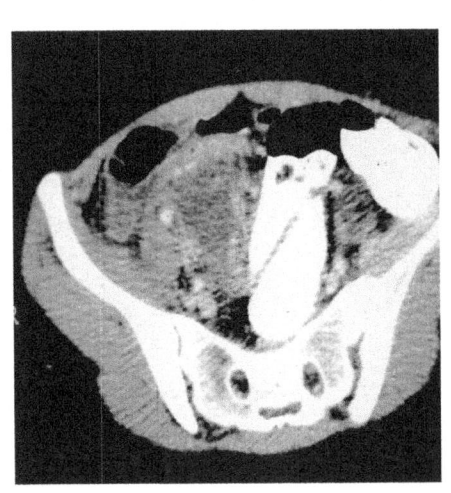

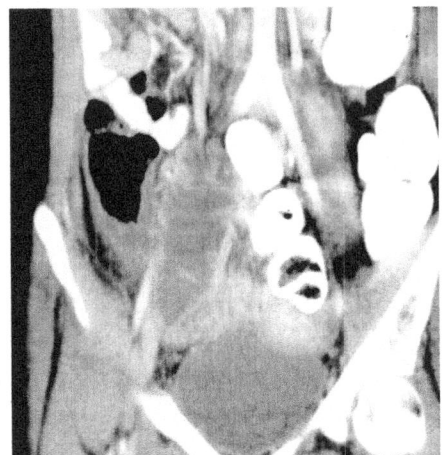

Questions

1. What are the findings seen in this scan?

2. What is the diagnosis?

3. What are the other complications that could happen in his case?

Answers and Discussion

The images show an ill-defined area of fluid collection in the right iliac fossa. The collection has thick irregular wall with peripheral enhancement on contrast administration. These findings are consistent with an appendicular abscess.

Acute appendicitis has many complications. These complications include:

- Formation of an appendicular mass
- Perforation
- Formation of an appendicular abscess
- Generalized peritonitis

Acute appendicitis is the most common cause of acute abdomen. It can occur in any age group, but it is rare in infants and in people older than 80 years. It occurs most commonly in people in their 2nd and 3rd decade of life.

Patients with acute appendicitis usually present with acute central colicky abdominal pain that lasts for hours and then is shifted to the right iliac fossa where it become sharp and stabbing in nature. The abdominal pain is usually exacerbated by movement or cough. Other symptoms are fever, anorexia, loose bowel motions, and vomiting.

On examination, there is mild fever, right iliac fossa tenderness, rebound tenderness, and crossed tenderness (Rovsing's sign). The presence of high fever should raise suspicion and prompt a search for complications. Other signs and findings depend on the site of the appendix. White cell count is usually elevated, but it can be normal in some cases.

CT scan is a useful tool in diagnosing acute appendicitis and assessing its complications in difficult patients (for example obese patients) and when ultrasound is equivocal. Before contrast administration, CT scan can show the dilated appendix (more than 7 mm), appendicolithes, and the periappendicular fat stranding. After contrast administration, enhancement of the appendix wall can be seen.

In complicated cases, CT scan can visualize the appendicular abscess or the appendicular mass. If the appendix is perforated and generalized peritonitis occurred, then CT scan can show the dilated bowel loops and the air-fluid levels caused by the accompanying intestinal obstruction. Free fluid inside the abdomen can also be seen on CT scan.

31. AN OLD MALE WITH INTESTINAL OBSTRUCTION

A 65-year-old male presented with abdominal pain and distension associated with bile-stained vomiting and constipation. The following images were taken from his contrast-enhanced CT scan.

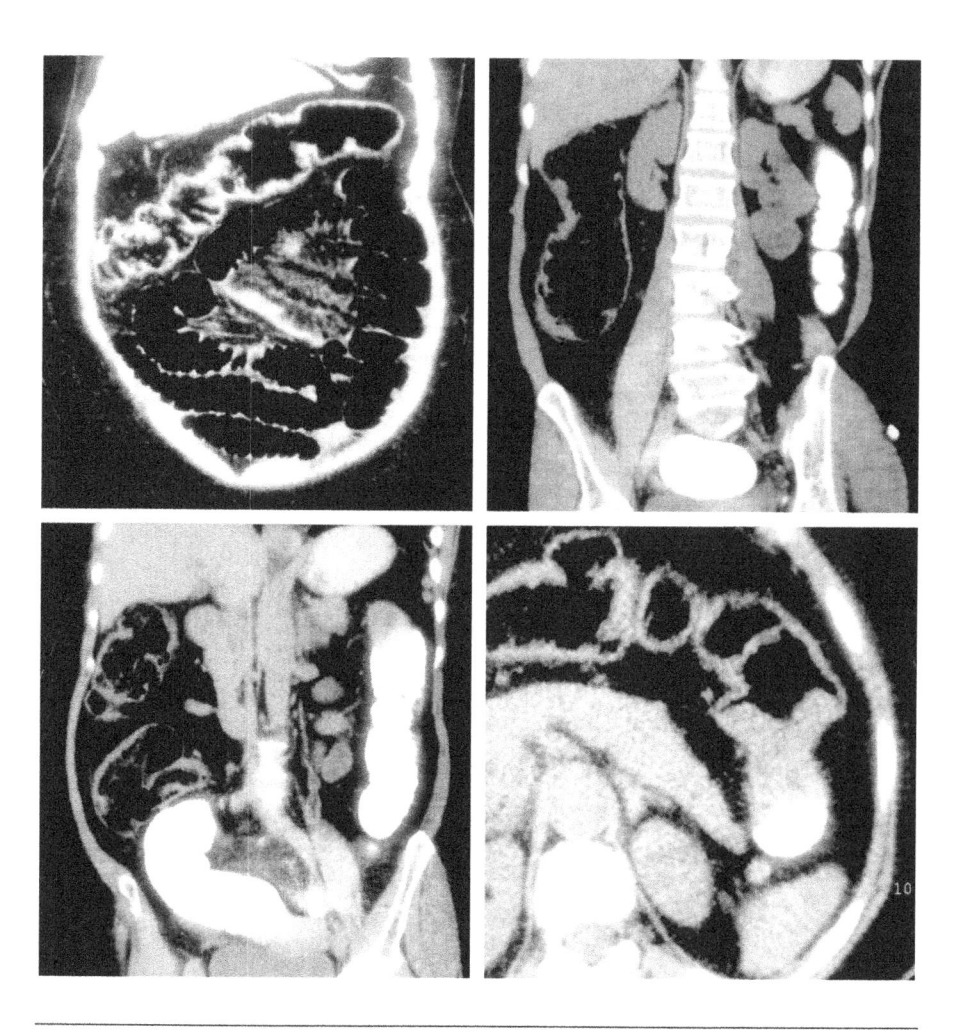

Questions

1. What are the findings seen in this scan?

2. What is the most likely diagnosis?

3. What are the predisposing factors for this condition?

Answers and Discussion

The images show dilatation of all small bowel loops and the caecum, ascending colon and transverse colon until the splenic flexure. Contrast material injected through enema doesn't pass through the splenic flexure of the colon. A colonic mass obstructing the lumen of the colon is seen at the splenic flexure with intact pericolic fat and no signs of invasion of the surrounding structures. The most likely diagnosis is bowel obstruction due to colonic carcinoma.

The predisposing factors for colonic carcinomas include:

- Family history of colorectal carcinoma.
- colon polyps (such as in familial adenomatous polyposis (FAP))
- Inflammatory bowel diseases (Ulcerative Colitis and Crohn's Disease).
- Diet high in fat and red meat and low in fibers, fruits and vegetables.
- Obesity and sedentary life style.

Colonic carcinoma is very common (it is the third most common malignancy affecting males and females in USA and UK). The most common age groups affected are people in their sixth to eighth decade.

The presentation of colonic carcinoma depends on the site of the tumor. Presentations include bowel obstruction, change in bowels habits, per rectal bleeding, and chronic iron deficiency anemia.

There are many systems for staging colonic carcinoma. These systems are TNM staging system, the Astler-Coller classification, and the Dukes classification. Prognosis depends on the stage of the carcinoma. 5-year survival can be as high as 95% for stage I tumours and as low as 10% for people with stage IV metastatic tumours. The most common sites of metastasis of colonic carcinoma are liver, lungs, and bone.

There are multiple choices for screening patient who are at risk for colonic carcinomas. Some of these options are Guaiac-based fecal occult blood test, Fecal immunochemical test, Flexible sigmoidoscopy, Colonoscopy, and CT colonography (virtual colonoscopy).

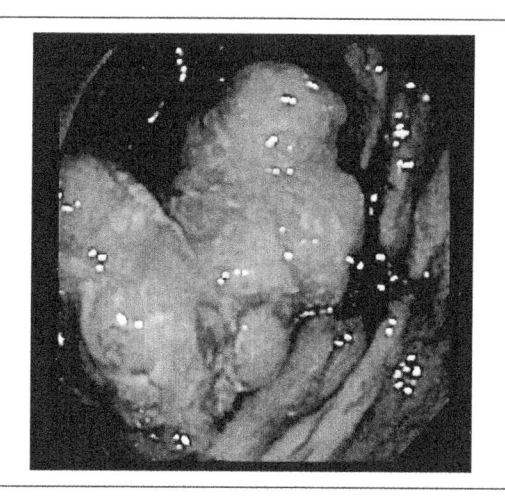

Endoscopy image of colon adenocarcinoma in sigmoid colon

(Original photo by Jiri.pekhart~commonswiki modified by Dcoetzee. Licensed under CC BY-SA 3.0.)

32. CYSTIC LESION IN THE PELVIS OF AN ADULT FEMALE

During a pelvic ultrasound study for a 28-year-old female a cystic lesion was found in the region of the left adnexa. The patient didn't complain from anything apart from mild lower abdominal discomfort. CT scan of pelvis was done with contrast. The images below are taken from the patient scan.

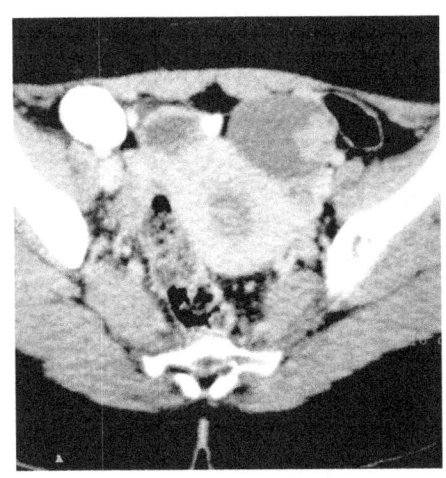

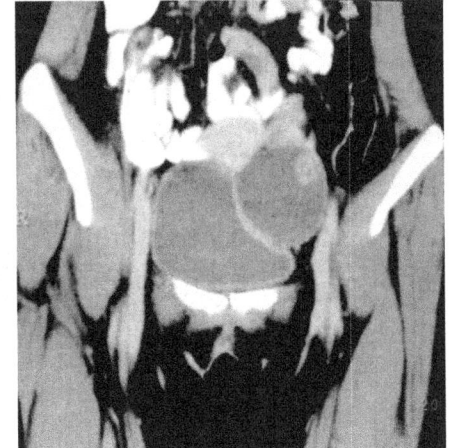

Questions

1. What are the findings seen in this scan?

2. What is the differential diagnosis of these finding?

3. What are the causes of this condition?

Answers and Discussion

The images show a cystic lesion with fluid density content in the region of the left adnexa. The lesion contains a mural nodule which has strong enhancement after contrast administration. These findings are consistent with a complex ovarian cyst.

Cystic lesions in the female pelvis can be ovarian or nonovarian in origin. The differentiation between the two types relies on identifying the normal ovaries and finding that the lesion is not related to them. Some of the most common types of cystic lesions in pelvis are listed in the table below.

Some of the most common cystic lesion found in female pelvis	
Ovarian	Nonovarian

• Functional cysts:
  ○ Follicular cysts
  ○ Corpus luteal cysts
• Neoplastic cysts:
  ○ Cystadenoma
  ○ Cystadenocarcinoma
• Teratoma.
	• Peritoneal inclusion cyst
	• Paraovarian cyst
	• Mucocele of the appendix
	• Abscess
	• Hematoma

Ovarian cysts can be asymptomatic or can present with lower abdominal pain/discomfort. The cyst might cause symptoms related to compression on its surrounding such as frequent micturition, tenesmus or discomfort with intercourse. When ovarian cysts produce hormones, they can present with precocious puberty or hirsutism.

When an ovarian cyst is found, it is important to look for signs that suggest malignancy in it. Features that can suggest malignancy of an ovarian cystic lesion include:

- Septations:
    o Thick septations.
    o Multiple septations.
- Wall:
    o Mural nodule.
    o Papillary projections.
- Contents:
    o Solid contents.

Even benign ovarian cysts can cause problems and present with complication. The most common complications seen are torsion of ovaries and rupture of the cysts.

33. BACK PAIN AFTER A TRAUMA

A 53-year-old female with a fall down had a CT scan done for her lumbosacral spine and for the lower part of her thoracic spine. The images below are taken from her CT scan.

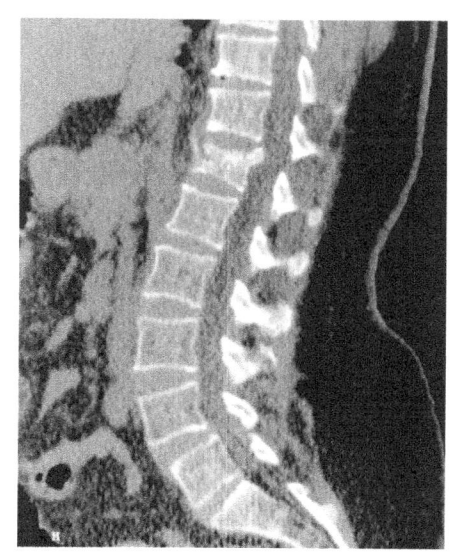

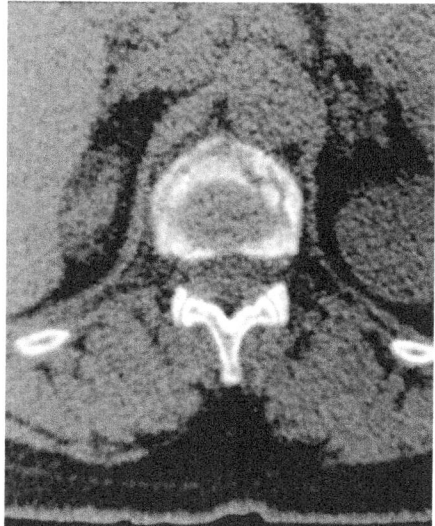

Questions

1. What are the findings seen in this scan?

2. What is the diagnosis?

3. What are the causes of this condition?

Answers and Discussion

The images show diffuse decrease in the bone density of lower thoracic and lumbar spine with compression of the body of T_{12} vertebra and no displacement of fragments, narrowing of spinal canal or affection of the posterior column at the level of T_{12} vertebra. These findings are consistent with anterior compression (wedge) fracture of T_{12} vertebra and osteoporosis of spine.

Anterior compression fractures can present with acute localized back pain after a trauma or with insidious back pain in old osteoporotic patient. They might also cause kyphotic deformity or compress spinal nerves causing pain or paraestheia at the area of the distribution of the nerve. The most common sites for these fractures are mid- and lower thoracic vertebra and the upper lumbar spine. They usually involve the superior endplate. If the inferior endplate is involved with normal superior endplate, then that should raise suspicion of a pathological fracture.

There are four subtypes of compression fractures of the spine based on the endplates involved in the fracture. These types are described in the table below.

Subtypes of compression fractures of the spine	
Type	Description
Type A	In this type, the superior and inferior endplates are involved.
Type B	Here only the superior endplate is involved.
Type C	The inferior endplate is the only one fractured in this type.
Type D	The superior and inferior endplates are intact, but the anterior cortex of the vertebra is buckled.

There are many other types of fractures that can occur in the thoraco-lumbar spine. Those are:

- Thoracic/lumbar lateral compression fractures
- Thoracic/lumbar burst fracture
- Thoracic/lumbar facet–lamina fracture
- Thoracic/lumbar chance fracture
- Thoracic/lumbar fracture- dislocation

Each of these fractures has its own features and etiology. Some of these fractures can mimic anterior compression fracture and need to be considered in its differential diagnosis (such as burst fractures, Chance fractures and pathologic fractures due to tumors).

Burst fracture (Unstable compression fracture) is a comminuted fracture that occurs in the mid- and lower thoracic vertebra or in the upper lumbar vertebra. In this type of fractures, both superior and inferior endplates are involved and widening of pedicles is seen. Usually fragments are seen in the spinal canal due to posterior displacement.

Chance fracture (flexion-distraction injury) is a fracture that usually occurs between T_{11} and L_3 vertebra due to high velocity injury or fall. In this fracture, there is disruption of all three columns of the spine. This fracture is usually associated with injury of the spinal cord. On imaging, comminuted fracture with wedging of the vertebral body is seen and the interspinous distance is increased posteriorly with kyphosis and separation of the facet joints.

34. AN OLD MALE WITH PROSTATE ENLARGMENT AND BACK PAIN

An 81-year-old male complains of back pain for the last few months and has previous history of prostate enlargment was referred to the radiology department for a CT scan of his lumbosacral spine. The images below are taken from his CT scan.

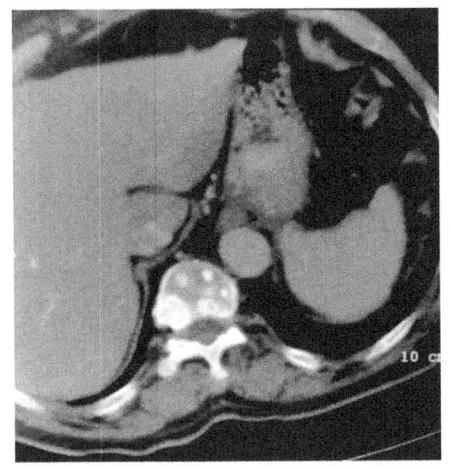

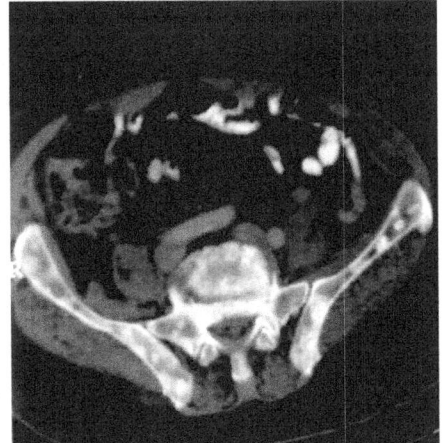

Questions

1. What are the findings seen in this scan?

2. What is the most likely diagnosis?

3. What are the differential diagnoses for these findings?

Answers and Discussion

The images show multiple well-defined hyperdense sclerotic lesions in the lumbar vertebrae and iliac bones. There are no signs of bone destruction or pathological fractures in the images, and no extension to soft tissues or compression on the spinal cord with narrowing of the spinal canal is seen. These findings are consistent with metastasis, and the source of the primary tumor is most likely to be a prostatic carcinoma according to the type of lesions and the history of the patient.

Focal lesions in spine can be classified into solitary lesions and multifocal lesions. Differential diagnosis of multifocal lesions in the spine includes:

- Metastatic tumor
- Myeloma/plasmacytoma
- Lymphoma and leukemia
- Hemangioma
- Bone island
- Pyogenic vertebral osteomyelitis
- Tuberculous vertebral osteomyelitis

Metastasis to the spine is very common. About third of the patients with metastatic tumours have metastasis to the spine. Most tumours that metastasize to the spine metastasize to thoracic spine, then lumbar spine. Cervical spine is the least common site for metastatic tumours in the spine. The most common sources of metastasis the spine are lung tumours and breast tumours, followed by gastrointestinal tract tumours, prostate tumours and lymphoma.

Most patients with spine metastasis are asymptomatic. When the symptoms appear, they are back pain, sensory or motor deficits or loss of control over bladder or bowel.

A common method of classification that is based on CT imaging and clinical findings and is used to guide the management of cases of spinal metastasis is the classification of Harrington which is explained in the table below.

\multicolumn{3}{c}{Harrington classification of spinal metastasis}
Class	**Description**	**Usual Management**
Class I	No significant neurologic involvement	Radiotherapy and/or chemotherapy
Class II	Involvement of bone without collapse or instability	
Class III	Major neurologic impairment (sensory or motor) without significant involvement of bone	
Class IV	Vertebral collapse with pain due to mechanical causes or instability but without significant neurologic compromise	Surgery
Class V	Vertebral collapse with pain due to mechanical causes or instability combined with major neurologic impairment	

Spinal metastasis can have variable appearances. It can be single or multiple lesions, well- or ill-defined. It can be osteolytic or osteosclerotic. The most common primary tumor that gives osteosclerotic metastasis is prostate carcinoma. Other less common malignancies include breast carcinoma, transitional cell carcinoma and carcinoid tumor.

35. AN OLD MAN WITH CHRONIC BACK PAIN

A 63-year-old male with chronic back pain had a CT scan of his lumbosacral spine. The images below are taken from his scan.

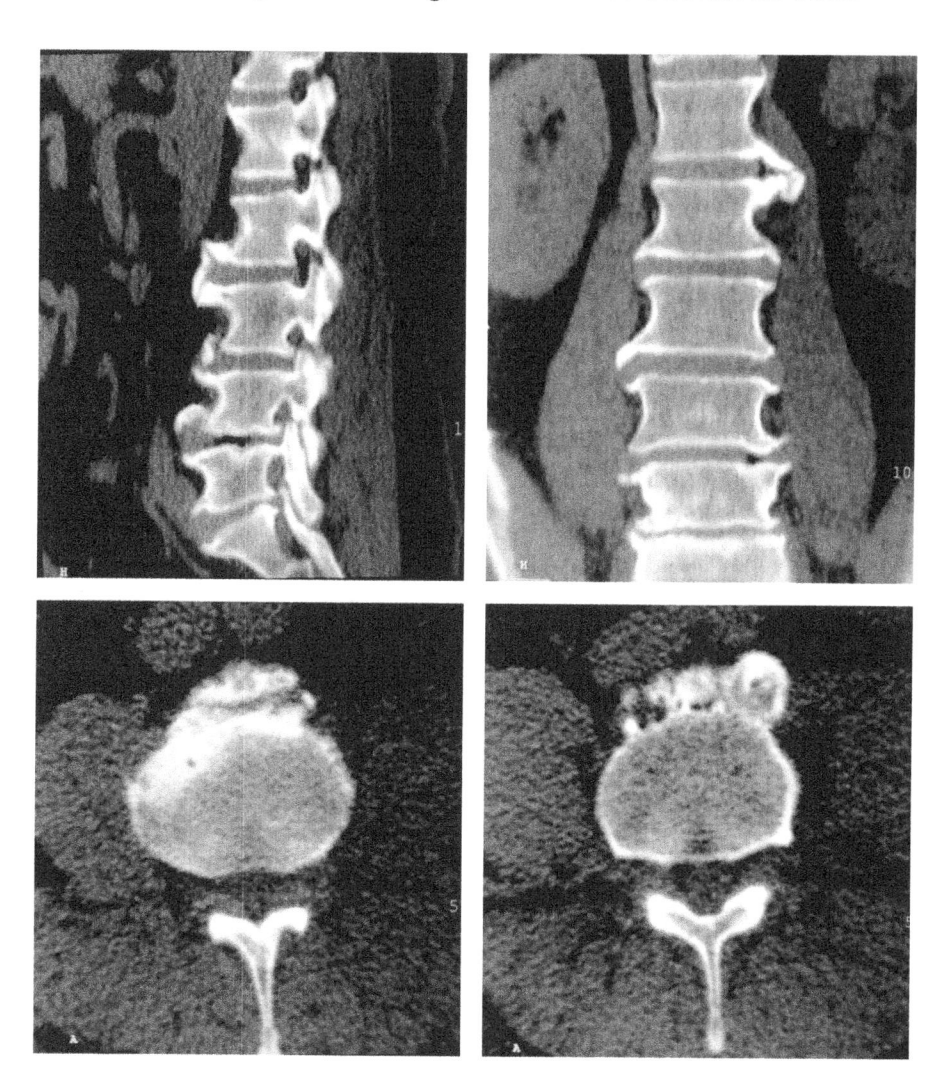

Questions

1. What are the findings seen in this scan?

2. What is the diagnosis?

Answers and Discussion

The images show loss of the lordotic curvature of the lumbosacral spine with osteophytes in multiple vertebrae and disc bulge with vacuum phenomenon in the intervertebral discs of L_{4-5}. These findings are consistent with spinal osteoarthritis (degenerative arthritis of the spine) with muscle spasm in the surrounding muscles.

Osteoarthritis is very common in many joints. Nearly all elderly patients have osteoarthritic changes in their spine when imaged and about 30% of people who are 30 years old or older have signs of osteoarthritis in their hands and about 33% of people who are 60 years old or older have signs of osteoarthritis of knee on imaging. Osteoarthritis can affect any joint, but it is most commonly seen in the weight-bearing joints. The most common features of osteoarthritis include:

- Narrow disc space
- Osteophytes formation
- Bone sclerosis

Risk factors for osteoarthritis include old age, genetic inheritance, congenital and developmental joints abnormalities, previous joint injuries, obesity, and activities that put recurrent stress on certain joints.

Osteoarthritis of spine has many presentations such as back or neck pain and stiffness, deformities, weakness of arms or legs, or paraestheia.

There are many complications of degenerative spinal diseases (including osteoarthritis of spine). The most important of these complications are:

- Spinal and foraminal stenosis
- Scoliosis and Kyphosis
- Segmental Instability

36. AN OLD FEMLAE WITH LOWER BACK PAIN AND STIFFNESS

A 64-year-old female with chronic low back pain and stiffness was referred for a CT scan of her lumbosacral spine. The images below are taken from her scan.

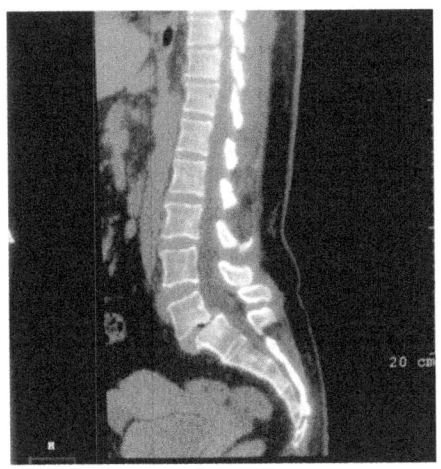

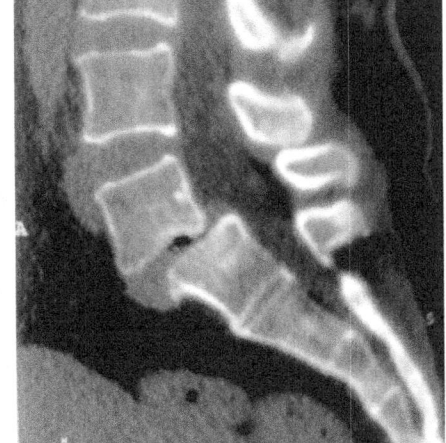

Questions

1. What are the findings seen in this scan?

2. What is the diagnosis?

3. What are the grades of this condition?

Answers and Discussion

The images show forward displacement of L5 vertebra over S1 vertebra. The displacement is between 25% to 50% of L5 vertebra. These findings are consistent with Grade 2 spondylolisthesis of L5.

Spondylolisthesis is graded according to the Meyerding classification which is explained in the following table and is illustrated in the figure on the following page.

Grade	Meyerding classification of Spondylolisthesis
	Description
Grade 1	In this grade, less than 25% of the upper vertebra has displaced forward over the lower one.
Grade 2	In this grade, between 26% and 50% of the upper vertebra has displaced forward over the lower one.
Grade 3	In this grade, between 51% and 75% of the upper vertebra has displaced forward over the lower one.
Grade 4	In this grade, between 76% and 100% of the upper vertebra has displaced forward over the lower one.
Grade 5	This grade is called spondyloptosis. In this grade, more than 100% of the upper vertebra has displaced forward over the lower one.

In spondylolisthesis, the upper vertebra moves forward over the lower vetebra. The most common site for spondylolisthesis is the lumbar spine. The most commonly affected lumbar veterbra is L5 (over S1).

There are many causes for spondylolisthesis. These causes are grouped in the Wiltse Classification. These causes lead to the classification of spondylolisthesis according to its cause into

Normal	Grade 1	Grade 2
Grade 3	Grade 4	

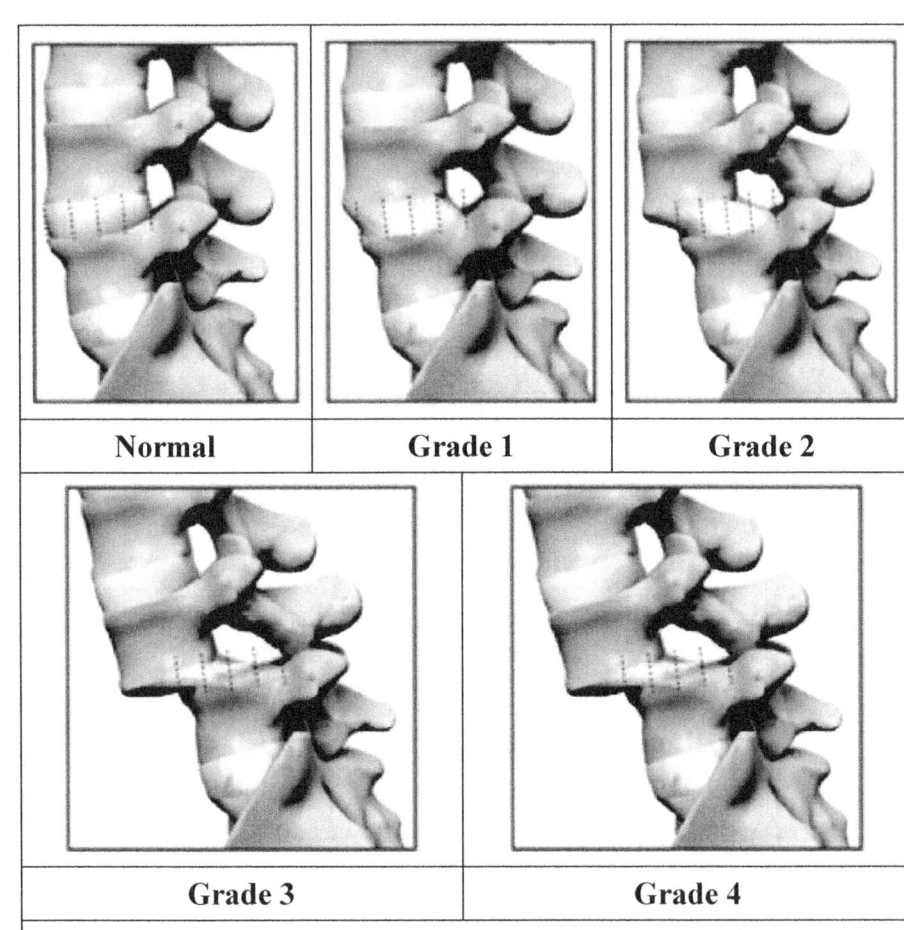

Grades of Spondylolisthesis

(This diagram is a derivative of "Spondylolisthesis stages" by Dr Harry Gkouvas, used under CC BY-SA 3.0. The modified diagram is licensed under CC BY-SA 3.0 by Dr Abdalla M. Gamal.)

dysplastic type (congenital), isthmic type (due to stress fracture or acute fracture), degenerative type, post-traumatic type, pathological type and iatrogenic type.

Forward movement of the vertebra can cause compression over the spinal cord or nerve roots leading to variable presentations. These presentations include pain and stiffness in the back or leg, paparaestheia in the back or leg, semi-kyphotic posture, and waddling gait.

CT scan is important in diagnosing spondylolithesis and in assessing its severity according to the Meyerding classification. The assessment of the condition severity is very important, because different grades of severity have different types of management. Many paitents with low grades can be managed conservatively.

INDEX

3

3rd ventricle 27, 30
3rd ventricle dilatation 26

4

4th ventricle 13, 30
4th ventricle dilatation 26

A

abdomen distension 93
abdominal distension 113
abdominal pain 80, 110, 113, 119
abdominal tenderness 99
Abnormal level of consciousness .. 38
abrasions 42
abscess 60, 68, 76, 108
Abscess 30, 118
Abscess formation 98
absent bowel sounds 99
acial injuries 42
acute abdomen 111
Acute appendicitis 111
Acute epigastric pain 97
Acute hemorrhage 7
Acute otitis media 60
acute otomastoidits 59
acute pancreatitis 98, 99
Acute phase 3
Acute Respiratory Distress
 Syndrome (ARDS) 99
acute sinusitis 51
Acute sinusitis 50, 56
acute stage 4, 76
Adenocarcinoma 80
adenoma 108
Adenoma 94

adnexa 117
aerobic bacteria 72
air fluid level 71
air-fluid level 60, 73
air-fluid levels 112
Airways compression 63
alcohol 99
alcoholic 97
alcoholics 10
allergic rhinitis 50
allergy 60
Allergy 53
Alpha-1-antitrypsin deficiency 84
alveolar effusion 81
alveolar process of the maxilla 43
ambient cistern 35
amoebiasi 72
amoebic liver abscess 91
Amoebic lung abscess 72
anabolic steroids 95
anaerobic bacteria 72, 76
aneurysms 6, 10
angle of the mandible 47
anorexia 110, 111
Anosmia 54
anterior compression fracture 122
anterior cranial fossa 39
antibiotic 73
antibiotics 54, 70
anticoagulant therapy 6, 10, 34
antihistamines 57
anti-leukotrienes 54
aphasia 3, 7
appendicolith 112
appendicular abscess 111, 112
appendicular mass 111, 112

115

appendix 112
appetite loss 66, 69
apraxia 7
aqueduct of sylvius 30
Aqueductal stenosis 30
arterial phase 94
arteriovenous malformation 34
arteriovenous malformations 6
arthritis 79
Arthritis 68
ascending colon 114
Aspergillus 51, 72
aspiration 71
aspiration pneumonia 72
Aspirin insensitivity 53
assault 42
assaults 46
Asthma 53
Astler-Coller classification 115
Astrocytomas 13, 14
ataxia 13, 18
AVM 10

B

back pain 125, 127, 129, 131, 133
Back pain 121
bacteria 51, 72, 91
bacterial cultures 76
Bacterial meningitis 35
bacterial pneumonia 84
Bacteroides 72
Balthazar et al. system for grading
 acute pancreatitis 100
basal ganglia 2
beaded appearance 83
benign intracranial cystic lesions ... 23
benign tumours 13, 14
berry aneurysm 34
bile-stained vomiting 113
biliary cystadenocarcinoma 92
Biliary Cystadenocarcinoma 90

Biliary Cystadenoma 90
Biliary Cystadenomas 91
Biloma 90
blasts injury 42
bleeding disorder 7
Bleeding from ear 39
Bleeding from nose 39
blood pressure 5
blunt trauma 39
body of the mandible 47
bone density 122
bone erosion 60
Bone island 126
Bone pain 80
Bone sclerosis 131
Botterell et al. scale 35
bowel obstruction 115
bowel perforation 31
Brain abscess 17, 50, 61
brain edema 18, 21, 38, 40
brain metastasis 18
brain tumours 21
breast 21
breast cancer 21
breast cancers 14
breast carcinoma 128
breast tumours 17
bronchial tree dilatation 83
bronchial tree obstruction 84
bronchiectasis 81
Bronchiectasis 83
bronchogenic carcinoma 79
Bronchogenic carcinoma 68
Bronchogenic cyst 68, 79
bruising inside the oral cavity 46
Bruising over ear or mastoid process
 39
brusies 42
bulging anterior fontanel 25, 28

C

caecum 114
calcification 20, 60, 78, 88, 107
Calcification 91
cancer of the head of pancreases .. 102
Candida 72
carcinoid tumor 128
Carcinoma 79
caudate nucleus 3
Cavernous sinus thrombosis 50
cavitary lesion 71, 81
cavitary lesions 67
Cavitary lesions 69
cavitations 66
central abdominal pain 110
central nervous system vessels 14
central scar 96
cerebellar hemisphere 13
Cerebellar metastases 14
cerebellopontine angle 24
cerebral cortex 20
Cerebral metastases 21
cerebral metastasis 17
Cerebrovascular accident 6
cerebrum 18
change in bowels habits 115
change in the level of consciousness
.... 28
cheeks 51
chest infection 77
chest pain 72, 74, 77, 80
chest trauma 76, 77
chest wall lipoma 87
chest x-ray 69
Chiari malformation 30
chills 74
choroid plexus 10
choroid plexuses 26
chronic back pain 129
chronic cough 66, 69
Chronic cough 82
chronic headache 12
Chronic hemorrhage 7
chronic iron deficiency anemia 115
Chronic nasal congestion 56
chronic otitis media 60
Chronic pancreatitis 99
chronic sinusitis 50, 51, 56
Chronic sinusitis 51
Circle of Willis 3
cirrhosis 95
cisterns 4
Clubbing 81
Cluster of grapes sign 91
CNS Infections 17
CNS lymphoma 17
CNS toxoplasmosis 17
CNS tumours 17, 28
coagulopathies 6
cocaine abuse 34
colicky abdominal pain 111
collapse of a lung 81
colon polyps 115
colonic carcinoma 114
colonic mass 114
Colonoscopy 116
colorectal carcinoma 115
column of Bertin 108
comminuted fractures 39
common bile duct 102
communicating hydrocephalus 26
communicatinghydrocephalus 27
complex ovarian cyst 118
compress spinal nerves 122
compression of CSF spaces 4
condyles of the mandible 46, 47
confusion 6, 7, 10
congenital cysts 24
Congenital deviation 56
Connective tissue disorders 56
connective tissues tumors 87
consolidation 67, 69, 75

constipation 64, 113
convlsions 16
convulsions . 6, 10, 18, 20, 24, 34, 38
Corpus luteal cysts 118
cortical grey matter 14
cough 66, 69, 70, 72, 77, 82, 84
cranial nerve dysfunction 13
cranial nerves injuries 40
crepitations 84
crepitiation 82
crescent shaped 10
crescent-shaped 9
Crohn's Disease 115
crossed tenderness 112
Cryptococcus neoformans 51
CSF absorption 26
CSF cleft sign 14
CSF leakage 39
CSF leakage from 39
CSF leakage from nose 39
CSF overproduction 26
CT colonography 116
Cullen sign 99
Curvularia 51
Cushing syndrome 80
Cylindrical bronchiectasis 84
cyst 68, 79
cyst rupture 119
Cystadenocarcinoma 118
Cystadenoma 118
Cystic bronchiectasis 85
cystic component 23
Cystic fibrosis 53, 84
cystic lesion 23, 117
Cystic liver lesion 89
cysts 23

D

Dandy-Walker malformation 30
daughter cysts 91
decreased hearing 58

deformities 131
degenerative arthritis of the spine 130
degenerative spinal diseases 131
degenerative spondylolisthesis 136
delayed phase 94
depressed skull fracture 38
depressed skull fractures 40
Depressed skull fractures 39
Dermoid cyst 23
Dermoid cysts 23, 24
deviation of the mandible 48
Diabetes 99
diabetes mellitus 103
diarrhea 91
difficult patients 112
dilatation in the bronchial tree ... 83
dilated appendix 112
dilated bronchi 83
dirty peripancreatic fat 98
disc bulge 130
discomfort with intercourse 119
dislocation 46
dislocation of the
  temporomandibular joint 46
displacement of fragments 46
Disseminated Intravascular
  Coagulation (DIC) 99
Draining 77
drowsiness 37
Dry mouth 56
Ductal adenocarcinoma 103
Dukes classification 115
dura 10, 21
dural base 14
dysmetria 13
Dysphagia 64
dysplastic spondylolisthesis 135
dyspnea 63, 64, 99

E

ear pain 58, 60

early morning vomiting 12
Echinococcus alveolaris 24, 90
Echinococcus granulosus 24, 90
Echinococcus multilocularis 24, 90
ectodermal cells 24
edema 4
effacement of brain sulci 27
effacement of sulci 4
effusion 76, 81
Ehlers–Danlos syndrome 56
empyema 75, 76
encephalopathy 35
endotracheal intubation 71
enema 114
enlarged liver 89
enlarging head 28
Entamoeba histolytica 91
entrapment 24
Epidermoid cyst 23
Epidermoid cysts 23, 24
Epidural abscess 50
Epidural hemorrhage 9
epigastric mass 93
epigastric pain 89, 97, 99
epistaxis 57
ERCP 99
ethmoid bones 43
ethmoid sinus 53
Eustachian tube 60
exertional dyspnea 63
external auditory canal 48
extraaxial 9, 13, 23
extraaxial cyst 23
Extraaxial hemorrhages 9
extraaxial location 14
extraaxial tumours 14
Extracranial complications 61
extradural lipoma 88
exudative stage 76
eye lids 88

F

facial asymmtry 42
facial bones 41
facial nerve 24
facial pain 51, 52, 57
Facial pain 54
facial palsy 19
Facial palsy 61
facial trauma 43
facial weakness 7
fall 42
fall down 121
falls 46
familial adenomatous polyposis .. 115
fat stranding 112
fat-density contents 23
Fecal immunochemical test 116
fecal occult blood test 116
fever 60, 70, 72, 77, 91, 99, 110, 111
Fever 74
fibrinopurulent stage 76
fibroblasts 77
fine needle aspiration 65
finger-like projections 17
Fisher Scale 35
fistula 60
flank pain 108
Flat cheecks 42
flattening of sulci 38
Flexible sigmoidoscopy 116
floating fractures 43
fluid collection 60, 75, 111
focal neurological deficit 18
Focal neurological deficit 38
focal neurological deficits 20
focal neurological signs 10
Focal nodular hyperplasia 94, 95
foetal lobulation 108
Follicular cysts 118
foramen of Monro agenesis 30
forehead 51

foreign body 84
foul smelling sputum 72
Foul smelling sputum 70
fracture of the nose 43
fractures of the mandible 45
fractures of the nose 46
frequent micturition 119
frontal horns of lateral ventricles 27
Functional cysts 118
fungal 51
fungal sinusitis 51
fungi 72
fusion of meninges 24

G

gallstones 99
gastrointestinal tract tumours 21
gastrointestinal tumours 17
generalized peritonitis 111, 112
genitourinary tumours 17
Glasgow coma scale 38
Glioblastoma multiform 20
Glioblastoma multiforme 17
Gliosarcoma 20
Goitre 64
Grey-Turner sign 99
grey-white matter interface 21
Guaiac-based fecal occult blood test
 116
guarding 99, 110
gunshot 42

H

Haemangioblastoma 13
Haemangioblastomas 14
Haemophilus 72
Haemophilus influenzae 60
hamartoma 79
head circumference 25
head trauma 33, 37, 41
headache 6, 10, 13, 18, 20, 24, 34, 57

Headache 54, 80
hearing impairment 58, 60
hearing loss 60
Hemangioma 94, 126
hematoma 38
Hematoma 118
hematuria 106, 108
hemianopia 3, 7
hemiparesis 3, 5, 7, 10
hemisensory loss 3
hemophilus influenzae 51
hemoptysis 69, 72, 84
Hemoptysis 80
hemorrhage 7, 20
hemorrhagic 6
hemorrhagic strokes 7
Hemorrhagic strokes 6
hemorrhagic transformation 4
hemosinus 42
Hepatic adenoma 94, 95
hepatic amoebiasis 72
Hepatocellular carcinoma 94
Hepatocellular carcinomas 95
hernias 31
high blood pressure 6
high fever 74, 112
hirsutism 119
HIV positive patients 17
hoarseness of voice 64
Hoarseness of voice 63
Hounsfield units 88
Hunt and Hess scale 35
Hydatid cyst 23, 79
Hydatid cysts 24, 90
hydrocephalus 26, 27, 29
hyperacute phase 4
Hyperacute phase 3
hypercalcemia 99
Hypercalcemia 80
hyperdense lesion 6
hyperlipidemia 99

Hypertension 5
hypertrophic pulmonary
　osteoarthropathy 81
hypertrophied nasal turbinates 51
hypertrophy of the nasal conchae .. 50
hypervascular metastases 95
hypodense basal ganglia 4
hypodense lesion 2
Hyponatremia 80
hypothyroidism 64
Hypovascular metastases 95
hypoxic-ischemic injury 35

I

iatrogenic spondylolisthesis 136
idiopathic 99
immunocompromised 72, 73
inability to speak 1
increase in head size 25
infants 28
infarction 2, 79
Infections 68
Infectious 79
inferior endplate 122
inflammation 76
Inflammatory 79
Inflammatory bowel diseases 115
infratentorial 13
insidious back pain 122
insula ribbon sign 4
insular cistern 35
interhemispheric fissure 35
intermediate stage 76
internal capsule 3
internal carotid artery 3
intestinal obstruction 113
intraaxial cyst 23
Intraaxial hemorrhages 9
intraaxial mass 20
intraaxial tumours 13, 14
intracerebral clots 36

intracerebral hemorrhage 6
intracerebral hemorrhages 6
Intracranial complications 50, 61
intracranial hemorrhage 9, 38, 40
intracranial hemorrhages 8
Intracranial hemorrhages 9
intracranial pathologies 10, 23
intracranial tumours 14
Intraductal papillary mucinous
　neoplasms (IPMNs) 103
intraglandular lipoma 88
intramuscular lipoma 88
intraparenchymal 10
Intraparenchymal hemorrhage 9
intraventricular clots 36
Intraventricular haematoma 30
intraventricular hemorrhage 9
Intraventricular hemorrhage 9, 10
iron deficiency anemia 115
irregular thin wall 71
irritability 60, 64
Ischemic 6
Ischemic strokes 3
isthmic spondylolisthesis 136

J

jaundice 80, 99
jaw 45
Jin et al. Grading 57

K

Kartagener syndrome 84
Klebsiella 72
Kyphosis 131
kyphotic deformity 122

L

Labyrinthine fistula 61
Labyrinthitis 61
laceration 48
lacerations 42

large head	25
Large-cell carcinoma	80
late stage	77
lateral ventricle	2
lateral ventricles	9, 30
lateral ventricles dilatation	26
Le Fort fractures	43
Le Fort I fractures	43
Le Fort II fractures	43
Le Fort III fractures	43
left middle cerebral artery	2
Lenticulostriate arteries	2
lentiform nucleus	4
lethargy	64
leukemia	126
leukocytosis	110
limbs weakness	1
limited mouth opening	48
linear fracture	38
Linear skull fractures	39
lines of fusion	24
Lipoblastoma	87
lipoma	87
Liposarcoma	87, 88
live functions	93
live metastasis	102
Liver abscess	90
liver cirrhosis	95
liver cyst	89
lobulated	23
locked mandible	48
loose bowel motions	111
lordotic curvature	130
loss of appetite	77
loss of consciousness	10, 34
loss of control over bladder or bowel	127
loss of grey-white matter differentiation	4
loss of sensation	7
loss of the ability to speak	6
low hemoglobin	7
lower abdominal discomfort	117
lower abdominal pain	119
lumbosacral spine	121, 130
lung	69
lung abscess	71, 73
Lung abscess	68, 79
lung abscesses	72
lung cancer	14, 21, 73, 80
lung carcinoma	17
Lung cavitations	66
lung collapse	81
lung cysts	69
lung fibrosis	86
Lung infarction	79
lung malignancies	69
lung nodule	78
lung tumours	17
Lymphoma	79, 126

M

Malformation	30
Malignancies	68
Malignant mesothelioma	76
Malignant pleural effusion	76
malnutrition	72
Mal-occlusion of the mouth	46
mandibular fractures	42, 47
Marfan syndrome	56
mass effect	2
mass in the flank	108
masses	69
mastoid air cells	59, 60
mastoid process	39
mastoiditis	59
Mastoiditis	61
maxilla	43
maxillary fractures	42
maxillary sinus	42
maxillary sinuses	50
maxillofacial fracture	42

measles pneumonia 84
Medullary carcinoma 108
medulloblastomas 14
Medulloblastomas 13
meninges 13, 39
meningioma 13
meningiomas 13
Meningiomas 13
meningitis 25, 39
Meningitis 35, 50, 61
mesothelioma 76
metastases 21
Metastases 13, 68, 94
metastasis 102, 126
Metastasis 17, 79, 126
Metastatic deposits 20
Metastatic tumor 126
Metastatic tumours 17
Meyerding classification 134
middle cerebral artery 3
middle cerebral artery occlusion 4
middle cranial fossa 23, 39
middle ear cavity 59, 60
middle ear infection 60
middle ear ossicles 60
midface 43
midline 23
midline shift 4
mild fever 110
mobile soft tissue masses 87
Moraxella catarrhalis 60
motor deficit 127
motor symptoms 3
motor vehicle accident 41, 42
motor vehicle accidents 46
Mucocele formation 50
Mucocele of the appendix 118
mucosal thickening 50, 51
mucous-containing diarrhea 91
multifocal lesions in the spine ... 126
multiloculated cyst 91

multinodular goiter 63, 64
Multiple septations 119
Mumps 99
mural nodule 118
Mural nodule 119
mural nodules 90
muscle spasm 130
Myeloma 126
myxedema 64

N

Narrow disc space 131
nasal bone 43
nasal bone fractures 42
nasal cavity 53
nasal conchae 50
nasal congestion 49, 51, 55, 56
nasal decongestants 57
Nasal deviation or depression 42
nasal discharge 51
nasal obstruction 49
nasal septum deviation 56
nasal steroid sprays 57
nasal stuffiness 51, 52
nausea 99
neck pain 34, 131
neck swelling 62, 64
Necrosis of the pancreas 99
Neoplastic 79
Neoplastic cysts 118
Neurocysticercosis 17
night fever 66, 69
night sweats 66, 69, 70, 74
nodular enhancement 94
nodule 78, 79, 81
nodules 64, 69
non-communicating hydrocephalus
.... 27, 30
non-obstructive hydrocephalus 26
nonovarian cysts 118
Non-small-cell lung cancer 80

nose	51
nystagmus	13

O

obese patients	112
obstruction of airways	42
obstruction of bronchial tree	84
obstructive hydrocephalus	27, 30
obstructive jaundice	101
obstructive lung disease	84
occipital horns of lateral ventricles	27
OCP	99
old hemorrhage	7
Oligodendroglioma	20
oncocytoma	108
open bite	48
open skull fracture	38, 40
oral contraceptive pills	95
Orbital abscess	50
Orbital cellulitis	50
orbits	50, 51
organizing stage	77
osteoarthritis	130
osteolytic	128
osteomyelitis	126
Osteomyelitis	50
osteophytes	130
Osteophytes formation	131
osteoporotic patient	122
osteosclerotic	128
otitis media	59, 60
otomastoidits	59
ovarian cysts	118
ovarian torsion	119
Overdrainage	31

P

pain	122
painless hematuria	106
Painless obstructive jaundice	101
palate	43
palpable mass in the flank	108
palpitation	64
palsy	24
pancreas	98
Pancreatoblastomas	103
paparaestheia	136
Papillary projections	119
paraestheia	122, 131
paranasal sinuses	53
paraneoplastic syndrome	80
Paraovarian cyst	118
parasellar region	23
paravertebral abscesses	76
pathological fracture	122
pathological fractures	46, 80
pathological spondylolisthesis	136
penis	88
Peptostreptococcus	72
per rectal bleeding	115
Perforation	111
periappendicular fat stranding	112
pericolic fat	114
perifocal edema	17
Periorbital ecchymosis	39
peripancreatic fat	98
peripheral enhancement	91
peripheral nodular enhancement	94
Peritoneal inclusion cyst	118
peritonitis	111
Persistent foetal lobulation	108
Petrositis	61
phlegmon	100
pituitary apoplexy	34
plasmacytoma	126
pleural cavity	76
pleural effusion	76
Pleural lipoma	87
pleuritic chest pain	72, 74, 77
Pleuritic chest pain	80
pneumonia	67, 69, 70, 76, 77, 81, 84
pneumothorax	67

polycystic liver disease 90
polyp 50
polypoidal mucosal thickening 50
polypoidal soft tissue masses 53
polyps 51
poor eration 60
poor feeding 60
positional dyspnea 63
Postauricular abscess 61
posterior cranial fossa .. 13, 20, 23, 31
posterior cranial fossa tumours 14
Posthemorrhagic 28
Postinfectious 28
post-resuscitation anoxic
 encephalopathy 35
post-traumatic spondylolisthesis .. 136
precocious puberty 119
Preseptal cellulitis 50
primary brain tumours 13
primary intraventricular hemorrhages
 10
primary tumours in the cerebellum 14
productive cough 70, 84
Progressive nasal stuffiness 53
Prominent column of Bertin 108
prostate carcinoma 128
prostate enlargment 125
prostatic carcinoma 126
pruritus 103
pseudocyst formation 31
Pseudocyst formation 98
pseudo-subarachnoid hemorrhage . 35
Pseudotumours 108
pterygoid processes 43
pulling of ear 60
pulmonary nodule 79
Pulmonary Tuberculosis 68
Pupils 42
pus 76
pyogenic liver abscess 91

Pyogenic vertebral osteomyelitis
 126
pyramidal fractures 43

Q

quadrigeminal cistern 26

R

raised intracranial pressure 20, 24
rebleeding 7
rebound tenderness 112
recurrent acute pancreatitis 99
recurrent artery of Heubner 3
recurrent convulsions 16
recurrent ear pain 60
recurrent sinusitis 56
Renal abscess 108
Renal adenoma 108
Renal cell carcinoma 108
Renal oncocytoma 108
René Le Fort 43
restricted movement of the mandible
 48
retrosternal extension 65
Rheumatoid arthritis 79
Rheumatoid Arthritis 68
rhinorrhea 52
Rhinorrhea 53
rhinovirus 51
rhonchi 82, 84
right iliac fossa tenderness 112
Right illiac fossa 110
Right illiac fossa pain 110
right upper quadrant pain 91
ring enhancement 17
Rovsing's sign 112
rubbing of ear 60

S

saccular bronchiectasis 85
Sarcoidosis 79

scalp hematoma 38
sclerotic lesions 126
Scoliosis 131
Secondary intraventricular
　hemorrhage 10
Segmental Instability 131
semi-kyphotic posture 136
sensory deficit 127
sensory loss 5
sensory symptoms 3
septations 90, 91
Septations 119
Serous cystadenoma of the pancreas
　.. 103
serous stage 76
sharp pain 110
shift of the midline 9, 13
shortness of breath .69, 72, 77, 82, 84
Shortness of breath 80
shunt 29, 31
Shunt infection 31
Shunt obstruction 31
Sigmoid sinus thrombosis 61
Simple cysts 90
Sinonasal polyposis 53
skull 43
skull base 43
skull base fracture 38
Skull base fractures 39
skull bones 18, 21
skull fracture 38
skull fractures 40
skull sutures 28
skull x-ray 43
Sleep disturbance 56
small bowel loops 114
small cell lung carcinoma 16
Small-cell lung cancer 80
smoking 80
snake venoms 99
snoring 55, 57

soft tissue debris 60
solid component 90
Solid contents 119
solitary lung nodule 78
solitary metastasis 18
solitary nodule 81
solitary pulmonary nodule 79
speculated irregular margins 81
spheniodal branch 3
Spinal and Foraminal Stenosis 131
Spinal osteoarthritis 130
Spindle cell lipoma 87
split pleura sign 75
spondylolisthesis 134
Spontaneous hemorrhage 21
Spontaneous intracranial hypotension
　.. 35
Spontaneous subarachnoid
　hemorrhage 34
sport injuries 46
sport injury 42
sputum 70, 72
Squamous cell carcinoma 80
stabbing pain 110
Staphylococcus 72
Staphylococcus aureus 51, 76
steroids 54, 99
stiffness 131, 133, 136
Streptococci 76
Streptococcus milleri 76
streptococcus pneumonia 51
Streptococcus pneumoniae 60, 76
stress fracture 136
stridor 80
Stroke 6
Subacute hemorrhage 7
subacute infarcts 4
Subacute phase 3
subarachnoid cyst 23
Subarachnoid cysts 23
subarachnoid hemorrhage 10, 34

Subarachnoid hemorrhage 9
subarachnoid hemorrhages 6
Subconjuncival hemorrhage 42
Subconjunctival hemorrhage 39
subcortical areas 20
subcutaneous lipoma 87, 88
subcuteneous mass 86
subdiaphragmatic abscess 76, 77
Subdural abscess 50
Subdural hematoma 31
subdural hemorrhage 9, 10
Subdural hemorrhage 9
submucous lipoma 88
Subperiosteal abscess 50
subperiosteal lipoma 88
subserous lipoma 88
subsynovial lipoma 88
subtotal opacification 53
sulci 33
superior endplate 122
Superior vena cava compression 64
suprasellar area 24
supratentorial 20
supratentorial mass 20
surface epithelium 24
surgical correction 57
swelling 46

T

TB cavitations 73
Temporal abscess 61
temporal bones 60
temporal horns of lateral ventricles 27
temporomandibular joints 46
tenderness 46
tenesmus 119
Teratoma 118
thalamus 6
The mortality rate 7

The World Federation of
 Neurological Surgeons Scale
 (WFNS) 35
thick irregular wall 111
thick irregular walls 67
thick septations 88
Thick septations 119
thick wall 91
thoracentesis 76
thoracic empyema 76
thoracic spine 121
thrombolytic therapy 6
thunderclap headache 34
thyroid cancer 64
thyroid functions test 62
thyroid gland 64
thyrotoxicosis 64
TNM system 103, 108, 115
transitional cell carcinoma 128
transverse colon 114
trauma 10, 24
traumatic 34
tremors 64
triad 108
trigeminal nerve 24
Tuberculoma 17
Tuberculosis 68
Tuberculous meningitis 35
tuberculous pneumonia 67, 69, 84
Tuberculous vertebral
 osteomyelitis 126
tubular bronchiectasis 84
tumor 84
Tumour 30
tumours 10

U

Ulcerative Colitis 115
Ultrasonography 65
unconscious 8
upper abdominal pain 99

Upper abdominal pain 80
upper respiratory tract 60

V

vacuum phenomenon 130
Varicose bronchiectasis 85
varicose type bronchiectasis 83
venous phase 94
ventricles 4, 9
ventricular system 26, 27
Ventriculoperitoneal shunts 31
vermian syndrome 13
vestibule-cochlear nerve 24
viral infection 60
virtual colonoscopy 116
viruses 51
visual symptoms 3
vomiting 10, 12, 13, 18, 28, 34, 38, 80, 97, 99, 111, 113

W

waddling gait 136
weakness 5
weakness of arms or legs 131
weakness of limbs 6
wedge fracture 122
weight loss .. 66, 69, 70, 93, 103, 106
Wheeze 80
White cell count 112
white matter 14
WHO grading system for Goitre 65
Wiltse Classification 135
workplace accidents 46
World Health Organization (WHO) 64

Z

zygoma 43
zygomatico-maxillary fracture 42

Made in the USA
Coppell, TX
25 March 2020